Geriatric Assessment

Geriatric Assessment

Multidimensional, Multidisciplinary and Comprehensive

Editor

Darryl Wieland

MDPI • Basel • Beijing • Wuhan • Barcelona • Belgrade • Manchester • Tokyo • Cluj • Tianjin

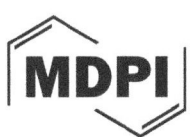

Editor
Darryl Wieland
Duke University Center for the
Study of Aging and Human Development
USA

Editorial Office
MDPI
St. Alban-Anlage 66
4052 Basel, Switzerland

This is a reprint of articles from the Special Issue published online in the open access journal *Geriatrics* (ISSN 2308-3417) (available at: https://www.mdpi.com/journal/geriatrics/special_issues/geriatric_assessment).

For citation purposes, cite each article independently as indicated on the article page online and as indicated below:

LastName, A.A.; LastName, B.B.; LastName, C.C. Article Title. *Journal Name* **Year**, *Volume Number*, Page Range.

ISBN 978-3-0365-0586-2 (Hbk)
ISBN 978-3-0365-0587-9 (PDF)

© 2021 by the authors. Articles in this book are Open Access and distributed under the Creative Commons Attribution (CC BY) license, which allows users to download, copy and build upon published articles, as long as the author and publisher are properly credited, which ensures maximum dissemination and a wider impact of our publications.

The book as a whole is distributed by MDPI under the terms and conditions of the Creative Commons license CC BY-NC-ND.

Contents

About the Editor vii

Preface to "Geriatric Assessment" ix

G. Darryl Wieland
New Variations on the Theme of Multidimensional Geriatric Assessment
Reprinted from: *Geriatrics* **2020**, *5*, 104, doi:10.3390/geriatrics5040104 1

Lucy Morse, Linda Xiong, Vanessa Ramirez-Zohfeld, Scott Dresden and Lee A. Lindquist
Tele-Follow-Up of Older Adult Patients from the Geriatric Emergency Department Innovation (GEDI) Program
Reprinted from: *Geriatrics* **2019**, *4*, 18, doi:10.3390/geriatrics4010018 5

Junko Ueshima, Keisuke Maeda, Hidetaka Wakabayashi, Shinta Nishioka, Saori Nakahara and Yoji Kokura
Comprehensive Geriatric Assessment and Nutrition- Related Assessment: A Cross-Sectional Survey for Health Professionals
Reprinted from: *Geriatrics* **2019**, *4*, 23, doi:10.3390/geriatrics4010023 13

Janine Overcash, Nikki Ford, Elizabeth Kress, Caitlin Ubbing and Nicole Williams
Comprehensive Geriatric Assessment as a Versatile Tool to Enhance the Care of the Older Person Diagnosed with Cancer
Reprinted from: *Geriatrics* **2019**, *4*, 39, doi:10.3390/geriatrics4020039 23

Tom Levett, Katie Alford, Jonathan Roberts, Zoe Adler, Juliet Wright and Jaime H. Vera
Evaluation of a Combined HIV and Geriatrics Clinic for Older People Living with HIV: The Silver Clinic in Brighton, UK
Reprinted from: *Geriatrics* **2020**, *5*, 81, doi:10.3390/geriatrics5040081 37

Katarina Wilhelmson, Isabelle Andersson Hammar, Anna Ehrenberg, Johan Niklasson, Jeanette Eckerblad, Niklas Ekerstad, Theresa Westgård, Eva Holmgren, N. David Åberg and Synneve Dahlin Ivanoff
Comprehensive Geriatric Assessment for Frail Older People in Swedish Acute Care Settings (CGA-Swed): A Randomised Controlled Study
Reprinted from: *Geriatrics* **2020**, *5*, 5, doi:10.3390/geriatrics5010005 49

Theresa Westgård, Katarina Wilhelmson, Synneve Dahlin-Ivanoff and Isabelle Ottenvall Hammar
Feeling Respected as a Person: a Qualitative Analysis of Frail Older People's Experiences on an Acute Geriatric Ward Practicing a Comprehensive Geriatric Assessment
Reprinted from: *Geriatrics* **2019**, *4*, 16, doi:10.3390/geriatrics4010016 67

Tahsin Barış Değer, Zeliha Fulden Saraç, Emine Sumru Savaş and Selahattin Fehmi Akçiçek
The Relationship of Balance Disorders with Falling, the Effect of Health Problems, and Social Life on Postural Balance in the Elderly Living in a District in Turkey
Reprinted from: *Geriatrics* **2019**, *4*, 37, doi:10.3390/geriatrics4020037 79

Katherine T. Ward, Mailee Hess and Shirley Wu
Geriatric Assessment in Multicultural Immigrant Populations
Reprinted from: *Geriatrics* **2019**, *4*, 40, doi:10.3390/geriatrics4030040 89

Lisa D Hobson-Webb, Paul J Zwelling, Ashley N Pifer, Carrie M Killelea, Mallory S Faherty, Timothy C Sell and Amy M Pastva
Point of Care Quantitative Assessment of Muscle Health in Older Individuals: An Investigation of Quantitative Muscle Ultrasound and Electrical Impedance Myography Techniques
Reprinted from: *Geriatrics* **2018**, *3*, 92, doi:10.3390/geriatrics3040092 . . . . **99**

Rebekah L. Young and David G. Smithard
The Clinical Frailty Scale: Do Staff Agree?
Reprinted from: *Geriatrics* **2020**, *5*, 40, doi:10.3390/geriatrics5020040 . . . . **113**

Antoinette Broad, Ben Carter, Sara Mckelvie and Jonathan Hewitt
The Convergent Validity of the electronic Frailty Index (eFI) with the Clinical Frailty Scale (CFS)
Reprinted from: *Geriatrics* **2020**, *5*, 88, doi:10.3390/geriatrics5040088 . . . . **119**

Gwendolen Buhr, Carrissa Dixon, Jan Dillard, Elissa Nickolopoulos, Lynn Bowlby, Holly Canupp, Loretta Matters, Thomas Konrad, Laura Previll, Mitchell Heflin and Eleanor McConnell
Geriatric Resource Teams: Equipping Primary Care Practices to Meet the Complex Care Needs of Older Adults
Reprinted from: *Geriatrics* **2019**, *4*, 59, doi:10.3390/geriatrics4040059 . . . . **125**

About the Editor

Darryl Wieland PhD, MPH; Senior Fellow, Duke University Center for the Study of Aging and Human Development. For the past 40 years, Dr. Wieland has conducted research on comprehensive geriatrics assessment and associated models of care, geriatrics education and workforce development, and program evaluation. In retirement, he presently serves as an investigative associate of the Geriatrics and Extended Care Data Analysis Center of the U.S. Department of Veterans Affairs.

Preface to "Geriatric Assessment"

Geriatric assessment—broadly defined—has become foundational to systems of care for frail elderly people at risk for functional decline, death, intensification of services, and long-term institutionalization. Its key feature is ascertainment of multiple dimensions of health and health risks—not only medical, but functional, cognitive, psychological, and socioeconomic factors. This multidimensionality is key to systematic screening and targeting using technologies to uncover frail, at-risk elderly people in their neighborhoods, homes, and at various other service contact points, for more intensive evaluation, i.e., "comprehensive geriatric assessment"—a multidisciplinary diagnostic and treatment process that identifies medical, psychosocial, and functional limitations of a frail older person to develop a coordinated plan to maximize overall health with aging. Care models embedding comprehensive and multidimensional assessment—in the community and in institutions—have been studied for years, with evidence supporting the efficacy of some in improving various care outcomes. In fact, early successes are partly responsible for the spread and differentiation of assessment-based programs, involving teams of specially trained health professions, together with the continued growth in the number of frail and at-risk elderly in demographically post-transition populations. From those earlier days, multidimensional geriatric assessment has come to support a variety of "co-care" or collaborative approaches with orthopedics, oncology, emergency medicine, surgery, and other medical disciplines. Now, developing countries are also rapidly aging and becoming wealthier, with improved health and social service resources. Thus, the interest in geriatric medicine and related care systems has been spreading, as well as the need to adapt and evaluate practice and assessment technologies in these new environments. The papers gathered in this Special Issue of Geriatrics all relate in some way to the foundational theme of multidimensional geriatric assessment, as they also exhibit the continuing evolution and differentiation of structures and processes of care built upon it. New technologies, populations, systems of care and financing, and workforce development strategies will need to hold true to these core principles.

Darryl Wieland
Editor

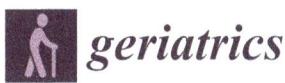

Editorial

New Variations on the Theme of Multidimensional Geriatric Assessment

G. Darryl Wieland

Duke University Center for the Study of Aging and Human Development, Durham, NC 27708, USA; gdw9@duke.edu

Received: 14 December 2020; Accepted: 15 December 2020; Published: 17 December 2020

Geriatric assessment—broadly defined—has become foundational to systems of care for frail elderly people at risk for functional decline, death, intensification of services, and long-term institutionalization. Its key feature is the ascertainment of multiple dimensions of health and health risks: not only medical, but functional, cognitive, psychological, and socioeconomic factors. This multidimensionality is key to systematic screening and targeting using technologies to uncover frail, at-risk elderly people in their neighborhoods, homes, and at various other service contact points, for more intensive evaluation, i.e., "comprehensive geriatric assessment", a multidisciplinary diagnostic and treatment process that identifies medical, psychosocial, and functional limitations of a frail older person to develop a coordinated plan to maximize overall health with aging [1].

Geriatric care models embedding comprehensive and multidimensional assessment—in the community and in institutions—have been studied for years, with evidence supporting the efficacy of some in improving various outcomes [2–4]. In fact, early successes are partly responsible for the spread and differentiation of assessment-based programs, involving teams of specially trained health professions, together with the continued growth in the number of frail and at-risk elderly people in demographically post-transition populations. This has been observed of geriatric assessment in other journal collections going back some decades [5,6]. From those earlier days, multidimensional geriatric assessment has come to support a variety of "co-care" or collaborative approaches with orthopedics, oncology, emergency medicine, surgery, and other medical disciplines. Now, developing countries are also rapidly aging and becoming wealthier, with improved health and social service resources. Thus, the interest in geriatric medicine and the related care system has been spreading, as well as the need to adapt and evaluate practice and assessment technologies in these new environments.

The papers gathered in this Special Issue of *Geriatrics* all relate in some way to the foundational theme of multidimensional geriatric assessment, as they also exhibit the continuing evolution and differentiation of structures and processes of care built upon it. Implemented or anticipated assessment-based models of "co-care" with other specialties, allied health providers, or for special clinical populations, are the subject of several reports [7–10]. One offering describes a protocol for a new experimental trial of comprehensive geriatric assessment in an acute care unit [11]; as person-centeredness is a common fundamental concern of clinicians and teams performing such assessments, it is fitting to have a second qualitative study on this topic from the same group [12]. Attention to common geriatric syndromes (e.g., falls) and assessment in developing countries and in multicultural immigrant populations is demonstrated in two other reports [13,14]. The use of technologies to more precisely assess the aspects of health of older patients toward the improvement of their care has been burgeoning in recent years, and is exemplified here by one contribution [15]. Finally, of great concern is the relative paucity of geriatrics professionals globally, weighed against the increasing need for them nearly everywhere. Numerous strategies have arisen to deal with these workforce and educational limitations, two of which are raised by the final papers in this Special Issue. First is the use of widespread screening and targeting by non-geriatrics professionals to identify older persons for further clinical assessment and associated care; the issue of how well these processes work is treated in the papers from Young and Smithard, and Broad et al. [16,17]. Buhr et al. evaluate the efficacy of direct transfers of geriatric assessment knowledge and skills from model geriatric resources teams to primary care practices [18].

Undoubtably, the papers appearing here represent only a small sampling of present activity, but they indicate the ongoing relevance of foundational principles as services and care for aging populations expand. New technologies, populations, systems of care and financing, and workforce development strategies will need to hold true to these core principles.

Funding: This research received no external funding.

Conflicts of Interest: The author declares no conflict of interest.

References

1. Rubenstein, L.Z.; Siu, A.L.; Wieland, D. Comprehensive geriatric assessment: Toward understanding its efficacy. *Aging Clin. Exp. Res.* **1989**, *1*, 87–98. [CrossRef] [PubMed]
2. Stuck, A.E.; Siu, A.; Wieland, D.; Rubenstein, L.Z.; Adams, J. Comprehensive geriatric assessment: A meta-analysis of controlled trials. *Lancet* **1993**, *342*, 1032–1036. [CrossRef]
3. Ellis, G.; Gardner, M.; Tsiachristas, A.; Langhorne, P.; Burke, O.; Harwood, R.H.; Conroy, S.P.; Kircher, T.; Somme, D.; Saltvedt, I.; et al. Comprehensive geriatric assessment for older adults admitted to hospital. *Cochrane Database Syst. Rev.* **2017**. [CrossRef] [PubMed]
4. Huss, A.; Stuck, A.E.; Rubenstein, L.Z.; Egger, M.; Clough-Gorr, K.M. Multidimensional preventive home visit programs for community-dwelling older adults: A systematic review and meta-analysis of randomized controlled trials. *J. Gerontol. Med. Sci.* **2008**, *63A*, 298–307. [CrossRef] [PubMed]
5. Rubenstein, L.Z.; Wieland, D.; Bernabei, R. Geriatric assessment technology: International research perspectives. *Aging Clin. Exp. Res.* **1995**, *7*, 157–158. [CrossRef] [PubMed]
6. Wieland, D.; Ferrucci, L. Multidimensional geriatric assessment: Back to the future (editorial). *J. Gerontol. Med. Sci.* **2008**, *63*, 272–274. [CrossRef] [PubMed]
7. Morse, L.; Xiong, L.; Ramirez-Zohfeld, A.; Dresden, S.; Lindquist, L.A. Tele-follow-up of older adult patients from the Geriatric Emergency Department Innovation (GEDI) Program. *Geriatrics* **2019**, *4*, 18. [CrossRef] [PubMed]
8. Ueshima, J.; Maeda, K.; Wakabayashi, H.; Nishioka, S.; Nakahara, S.; Kokura, Y. Comprehensive geriatric assessment and nutrition-related assessment: A cross-sectional survey for health professionals. *Geriatrics* **2019**, *4*, 23. [CrossRef] [PubMed]
9. Overcash, J.; Ford, N.; Kress, E.; Ubbing, C.; Williams, N. Comprehensive geriatric assessment as a versatile tool to enhance the care of the older person diagnosed with cancer. *Geriatrics* **2019**, *4*, 39. [CrossRef] [PubMed]
10. Levett, T.; Alford, K.; Roberts, J.; Adler, Z.; Wright, J.; Vera, J.H. Evaluation of a combined HIV and geriatrics clinic for older people living with HIV: The Silver Clinic in Brighton, UK. *Geriatrics* **2020**, *5*, 81. [CrossRef] [PubMed]
11. Wilhelmson, K.; Hammar, I.A.; Ehrenberg, A.; Niklasson, J.; Eckerblad, J.; Ekerstad, N.; Westgård, T.; Holmgren, E.; Åberg, N.D.; Dahlin Ivanoff, S. Comprehensive geriatric assessment for frail older people in Swedish acute care settings (CGA-Swed): A randomised controlled study. *Geriatrics* **2020**, *5*, 5. [CrossRef] [PubMed]
12. Westgård, T.; Wilhelmson, K.; Dahlin-Ivanoff, S.; Ottenvall Hammar, I. Feeling respected as a person: A qualitative analysis of frail older people's experiences on an acute geriatric ward practicing a comprehensive geriatric assessment. *Geriatrics* **2019**, *4*, 16. [CrossRef] [PubMed]
13. Değer, T.B.; Saraç, Z.F.; Savaş, E.S.; Akçiçek, S.F. The relationship of balance disorders with falling, the effect of health problems, and social life on postural balance in the elderly living in a district in Turkey. *Geriatrics* **2019**, *4*, 37. [CrossRef] [PubMed]
14. Ward, K.T.; Hess, M.; Wu, S. Geriatric assessment in multicultural immigrant populations. *Geriatrics* **2019**, *4*, 40. [CrossRef] [PubMed]

15. Hobson-Webb, L.D.; Zwelling, P.J.; Pifer, A.N.; Killelea, C.M.; Faherty, M.S.; Sell, T.C.; Pastva, A.M. Point-of-care quantitative assessment of muscle health in older individuals: An investigation of quantitative muscle ultrasound and electrical impedance myography techniques. *Geriatrics* **2018**, *3*, 92. [CrossRef] [PubMed]
16. Young, R.L.; Smithard, D.G. The Clinical Frailty Scale: Do staff agree? *Geriatrics* **2020**, *5*, 40. [CrossRef] [PubMed]
17. Broad, A.; Carter, B.; Mckelvie, S.; Hewitt, J. The convergent validity of the electronic Frailty Index [eFI] with the Clinical Frailty Scale [CFS]. *Geriatrics* **2020**, *5*, 88. [CrossRef] [PubMed]
18. Buhr, G.; Dixon, C.; Dillard, J.; Nickolopoulos, E.; Bowlby, L.; Canupp, H.; Matters, L.; Konrad, T.; Previll, L.; Heflin, M.; et al. Geriatric Resource Teams: Equipping primary care practices to meet the complex care needs of older adults. *Geriatrics* **2019**, *4*, 59. [CrossRef] [PubMed]

Publisher's Note: MDPI stays neutral with regard to jurisdictional claims in published maps and institutional affiliations.

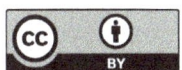

© 2020 by the author. Licensee MDPI, Basel, Switzerland. This article is an open access article distributed under the terms and conditions of the Creative Commons Attribution (CC BY) license (http://creativecommons.org/licenses/by/4.0/).

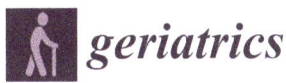

Article

Tele-Follow-Up of Older Adult Patients from the Geriatric Emergency Department Innovation (GEDI) Program

Lucy Morse [1], Linda Xiong [1], Vanessa Ramirez-Zohfeld [1], Scott Dresden [2] and Lee A. Lindquist [1,*]

1. Division of General Internal Medicine & Geriatrics, Northwestern University Feinberg School of Medicine, Chicago, IL 60611, USA; Lucy.Morse@northwestern.edu (L.M.); Linda.Xiong@northwesten.edu (L.X.); Vanessa-Ramirez-0@northwesten.edu (V.R.-Z.)
2. Department of Emergency Medicine, Northwestern University Feinberg School of Medicine, Chicago, IL 60611, USA; S-Dresden@northwestern.edu
* Correspondence: LAL425@NORTHWESTERN.EDU; Tel.: +1-312-695-4525

Received: 6 December 2018; Accepted: 24 January 2019; Published: 29 January 2019

Abstract: The objective of this study was to characterize the content and interventions performed during follow-up phone calls made to patients discharged from the Geriatrics Emergency Department Innovation (GEDI) Program and to demonstrate the benefit of these calls in the care of older adults discharged from the emergency department (ED). This study utilizes retrospective chart review with qualitative analysis. It was set in a large, urban, academic hospital emergency department utilizing the Geriatric Emergency Department Innovations (GEDI) Program. The subjects were adults aged 65 and over who visited the emergency department for acute care. Follow-up telephone calls were made by geriatric nurse liaisons (GNLs) at 24–72 h and 10–14 days post-discharge from the ED. The GNLs documented the content of the phone calls, and these notes were analyzed through a constant comparative method to identify emergent themes. The results showed that the most commonly arising themes in the patients' questions and nurses' responses across time-points included symptom management, medications, and care coordination (physician appointments, social services, therapy, and medical equipment). Early follow-up presented the opportunity for nurses to address needs in symptom management and care coordination that directly related to the ED admission; later follow-up presented a unique opportunity to resolve sub-acute issues that were not addressed by the initial discharge plan and to manage newly arising symptoms and patient needs. Thus, telephone follow-up after emergency department discharge presents an opportunity to better connect older adults with appropriate outpatient care and to address needs arising shortly after discharge that may not have otherwise been detected. By following up at two discrete time-points, this intervention identifies and addresses distinct patient needs.

Keywords: Emergency department; follow-up phone calls; older adults

1. Introduction

Providing affordable, quality health care to older adults in the emergency department (ED) is of paramount concern in the present and future medical landscapes. The number of adults ages 65 and over in the United States (US) is projected to more than double in the next 40 years, comprising nearly 25% of the total population by 2069 [1]. This older adult population is more likely to be admitted to the hospital following a visit to the emergency department relative to younger adults, and nearly half are readmitted within six months. Moreover, hospital admission is both costly and associated with a number of adverse outcomes for older patients, especially [2–4]. Several novel interventions have been designed to identify at-risk older adults interfacing with the emergency department in an effort to streamline impactful care and to reduce the financial and personnel burdens that accompany the hospital admission of older adults [5–7].

One such point of intervention is avoidable admission for reasons other than acute illness, including functional decline, polypharmacy, dementia, and an unstable living environment. Although these conditions may not be grounds for admission independently, in combination with acute illness and complex medical needs, they may lead to imminent risk to the patient if discharged [8,9].

1.1. The Geriatric Emergency Department Innovation (GEDI) Program

The GEDI program was developed to optimize the treatment of older adult patients entering the emergency department in order to shorten ED visits and reduce hospital admissions, while connecting patients with the social and outpatient medical services best suited to their needs [9]. At Northwestern Memorial Hospital (NMH), nurses specially trained in geriatrics—geriatric nurse liaisons (GNLs)—identify older adults through the Identify Seniors at Risk (ISAR) tool and perform further screens for common geriatric syndromes by assessing for cognition (Short Portable Mental Status Questionnaire), delirium (Confusion Assessment Method), functional status, (Katz Activities of Daily Living), fall risk (Timed Up and Go test), caregiver strain (Modified Caregiver Strain Index), and transition readiness (Care Transitions Measure-3) [9,10]. GNLs assess the patient and determine if the patient can receive optimal treatment at home with outpatient follow-up instead of being admitted to the hospital. Hospitalization is well-established to be detrimental for older adults with resulting decreased physical function, worsening cognition, medication issues, and a multitude of other adverse effects. Based on results from the GNL testing series, patients are referred to primary care and specialist services, physical therapy, occupational therapy, and social and home care services as appropriate. The GNL designs a care plan for discharge, and then, the patient is sent home from the ED. After discharge, the GNL makes follow-up phone calls at two time-points following the ED admission to assess the continuing needs in care and answer any medical or logistical questions that may have arisen since the ED discharge [9,10].

The results from NMH's GEDI program have shown that the intervention results in a significant decrease in the hospital admission of older adults presenting to the emergency department [9]. Individual components of the GEDI program's effectiveness and impact, however, remain to be analyzed. Specifically, the impact of the telephone follow-up care provided to patients discharged from the GEDI program and ED has yet to be examined.

1.2. Follow-Up in Emergency and Ambulatory Care Settings

Previous research on the impact of follow-up care in the medical setting strongly indicates its important role in high-value, low-cost care. Follow-up phone calls made by pharmacists 48 h after hospital discharge at an academic medical center resulted in greater patient satisfaction, medication resolution, and medical referral for a subset of patients and fewer ED readmissions 30 days post-discharge for patients receiving the phone calls [11]. Similar interventions in pediatric, geriatric, and adult populations have demonstrated that calls can present an opportunity to assist a significant proportion of patients with medical questions and issues arising post-discharge and can increase patient adherence to appointments and care instructions in post-discharge and traditional clinic settings [12–15]. While the value of follow-up phone calls in the setting of the GEDI program at NMH is strongly indicated, the outcomes of these calls remain unexamined. Furthermore, the value of these follow-up calls in addressing patient needs as it relates to timepoint post-discharge remains, to our knowledge, unstudied in the context of care for older adults.

The objective of this study was to characterize the content and interventions performed during follow-up phone calls made to discharged patients who presented at the GEDI program academic medical center and to demonstrate the benefit of these calls to the care of older adults discharged from the emergency department.

2. Materials and Methods

2.1. Participants

All the patients over the age of 65 presenting to the emergency room and meeting the ISAR criteria for further work-up through the GEDI program received the follow-up phone calls that were the subject of this analysis. The data were anonymized prior to qualitative analysis. This project was considered exempt by the Northwestern University Institutional Review Board.

2.2. Data Collection

GEDI follow-up phone calls were made at two time-points: 24–72 h and 10–14 days following the primary ED admission. The GNL responsible for the patient case performed the follow-up phone call and transcribed the conversation in an open-response format; notes from the patient charts were abstracted, and these notes were the subject of the data analysis, until saturation of themes was achieved.

2.3. Data Analysis

The transcripts were then de-identified and analyzed by 3 authors (LL, LM, and LX) using content and constant comparative techniques [16], through which the coders independently assessed the participant responses for focal themes. The authors then convened to compare and compile their findings to create a list of major themes, which were discussed through further meetings, such that a consensus was reached in all the cases of initial discrepancy. The coders independently organized the content into an overarching categorical system: Multiple coders were allowed to independently develop categorical systems in order to control for the subjective bias each coder brings to the analytic process [17]. From these overarching categories, the coders synthesized the relevant themes and compared them across time-points.

3. Results

3.1. Obtaining Thematic Saturation

The responses to telephone follow-up were consecutively abstracted and qualitatively analyzed, until thematic saturation was reached (e.g., consensus of the research team that no new information was emerging in the data collection) [18–20]. Hematic saturation was determined to be completed after 57 charts. Prior qualitative research has shown that as few as 8–12 interviews are needed to reach thematic saturation [21,22].

3.2. Subject Characteristics

For the 57 subjects, the mean age was 88.6 years (range 66–96 years). The subjects had a mean ISAR score of 4 (range 1–6). From a cognitive perspective, the subjects scored a mean 1.65 (range 0–7) on the Short Portable Mental Status Questionnaire (SPMSQ, normal is less than 2). From a functional perspective, of the six basic activities of daily living (ADLs: eating, bathing, getting dressed, toileting, transferring, and continence), the subjects were able to do a mean of 5.28 (range 0–6) independently without assistance. These data were self-reported. A total of 14 subjects used an assistive device (cane or walker) and scored a mean of 15.5 s (range 8–34 s) on the Timed Up and Go test.

3.3. Key Themes

Key themes in the patients' concerns and the nurses' responses emerged in both time-points. The emergent themes in the patient concerns included clinical symptoms, medication questions, medical equipment, therapy or home health services, and follow-up with specialists or primary care providers (Table 1). The emergent themes in the nurse responses included providing clinical information, medication counseling, care coordination relating to appointments, and communication with social workers to arrange other social services (Table 2). These themes were largely overlapping across time-points; however, certain themes were unique to the later time point, and notably, certain themes were much more frequently encountered in one time point or the other. Upon further investigation of frequency disparities in theme across the time-points, certain content specificities within the overarching categories were found to vary, leading to the demonstrated differences.

Table 1. Patient concerns at follow-up: Patient concerns arising 24–72 h and 10–14 days post-discharge.

Emergent Themes	Selected Quotes
Clinical/symptom management	"The patient discussed how long her eye might remain red...informed to follow-up with ophthalmologist or emergency department if increased discharge, draining, bleeding from the eye, pain, or visual disturbances."
Medication	"Taking acetaminophen only 2 times a day. Afraid of aggravating liver." "Did quiz him about the use of his insulin and he states that his blood sugars have been in the 130-150 range. States he is checking his sugars two times a day"
Therapy, home health, or medical equipment	"Patient concerned about being alone and having to take shower without having someone check on her" "Questions in regard to when home health care and physical therapy would come to evaluate the patient"
Physician follow-up	"Has appointment on the 23rd. Will be receiving home occupational therapy in addition to home physical therapy. Patient lost list of geriatric psychiatrists, asked to resend to home. Mailed today."
Transitions of care **	"Discharged home from skilled nursing facility on 4/18. Scheduled for blood draw and evaluation in the Coumadin Clinic today. Appointment with cardiologist scheduled for 4/29."

** Theme only present at the 10–14-day follow-up. Quotes edited for grammar and clarity.

Table 2. Nurse response at follow-up: nurses' responses to patient concerns identified at 24–72 h and 10–14 days post-discharge.

Emergent Themes	Selected Quotes
Symptom counseling	"Informed to elevate, apply ice or take Tylenol, as needed" "instructed on warm compresses and stretching"
Medication counseling	"Not discharged from emergency department observation unit with any pain medications. Encouraged acetaminophen 650 mg every 4 h as needed"
Physician care coordination	"Encouraged to follow-up with primary care physician (PCP) and Gastroenterologist as scheduled for increased pain" "... Physician referral services contacted and made appointment for patient for follow-up with primary care physician for Wednesday this week."
Therapy, home health, or medical equipment coordination	"Having difficulty obtaining walker, which was told was ordered two weeks ago, but home care agency said they are waiting on physician order. Will contact our social worker to help facilitate. 1445: Prescription obtained for walker from emergency department physician faxed by the Geriatric Emergency Department Innovation (GEDI) nurse liaison and will facilitate walker delivery to pt." "Patient required multiple calls to help facilitate outpatient physical therapy. Prescription faxed to rehabilitation center with diagnosis."
Social work/services coordination	"...To have endoscopy and colonoscopy at the end of May. Looking into Medical Alert Systems. Given several names from Social worker list."
Caregiver coordination **	"Patient states he is not aware of visits; caregiver daughter is in charge. Called daughter and left a message if she needs any assistance with appointment scheduling."

** Theme only present at 10–14-day follow-up. Quotes edited for grammar and clarity.

3.4. Comparison across Timepoints

3.4.1. Clinical Symptoms

Clinical symptoms made up a large portion of issues discussed at both the 24–72-h and 10–14-day time-points; however, the concerns differed in content within this theme. Clinical concerns raised shortly after discharge were typically found to relate to the concern for which the patient presented to the ED initially, as exemplified by this follow-up note: *"The patient discussed how long her eye might remain red...informed to follow-up with ophthalmologist or ED if increased discharge, draining, bleeding from the eye, pain, or visual disturbances."* By contrast, symptom-related concerns at 10–14 days were sometimes unrelated to the cause for ED admission, as shown by this note: *"Has an appt. with primary care physician in another week. I asked her to speak with the doctor about her elevated blood pressure. Patient was concerned that it has not been controlled with her current medication but will seek guidance from primary care physician."* A subset of clinical concerns presenting at the 10–14-day time-point was entirely unrelated to the chief concern at the ED admission: *"Complaining of productive cough and occasional wheezing. Using inhaler with some relief"*. By contrast, none of the clinical concerns identified at 24–72 h were entirely new or unrelated to the concern precipitating the ED visit. In short, while clinical/symptom-related concerns were a common feature of the follow-up calls at both time-points, the later time-point demonstrated use in identifying sub-acute or unrelated clinical concerns that had not been apparent at the earlier time-point.

3.4.2. Physician Follow-Up Appointment Scheduling

Although follow-up physician scheduling was managed at both time-points, concerns and new information were more frequently elicited at the later time-point; while instructions were given to follow up and appointments were scheduled by the GNLs at the earlier time-point, the later time-point allowed the nurses to follow up on planned/recommended appointments that had not successfully been made, as shown in this note: *"Spoke with patient to verify that she called the ophthalmology clinic for an appointment...notified her that I would call back tomorrow to be sure she was ok and had made her follow-up appt...addendum: scheduled follow-up ophthalmology appointment for 4/23/13 at 1500."*

3.4.3. Durable Medical Equipment (DME), Physical Therapy (PT), and Home Health Nursing (HN) Coordination

Nurse coordination of durable medical equipment (DME), physical therapy (PT), and home health nursing (HN) took place more frequently at the 24–72-h follow-up relative to the 10–14-day follow-up. Early communication is critical for quick access to DMEs and HN services, such as home safety evaluations: *"Having difficulty obtaining walker, which was told was ordered 2 weeks ago, but home health agency said they are waiting on physician order. Will contact our social worker to help facilitate. 1445: Prescription obtained for walker from emergency department physician, faxed by the Geriatric Emergency Department Innovation (GEDI) nurse liaison and will facilitate walker delivery to patient."*

However, calls at the second time-point added value in that they allowed nurses to connect patients with services that were identified as potentially beneficial upon the initial physician follow-up, as shown here: *"The patient states her primary care physician suggested physical therapy. Will call office to see about order for physical therapy."*

4. Discussion and Conclusions

This study set out to characterize the content and interventions performed during follow-up phone calls made to discharged patients who presented at the GEDI program academic medical center and to demonstrate the potential benefit of these calls to the care of older adults discharged from the emergency department. Qualitative analysis revealed key emergent themes in both the patient concerns expressed during the calls, as well as the nurse responses to the patient needs raised during in the follow-up. Concerns regarding clinical symptoms, medications, specialist and primary care physician follow-up, and durable medical equipment, physical therapy, and home health nursing services arose frequently across both time-points. The nurses responded to such concerns by providing clinical symptom and medication counseling, confirming or scheduling physician follow-up appointments and interfacing with case managers in order to navigate patient access to durable medical equipment, physical therapy, and home health nursing services; these actions were taken by nurses at both time-points. Some patient concerns and nurse responses were only encountered at the later time-point, including caregiver coordination and management of transitions of care.

4.1. Significance of Cross-Timepoint Comparisons

While there was a great amount of consistency across time-points where the emergent themes were concerned, a variation of content within themes, as well as differences in frequency of theme presence across time points, was identified. Clinical concerns and symptom management at the 24–48-h time-point was consistently related to the chief concern that precipitated the ED intake, while this theme at the 10–14-day follow-up included newly identified clinical concerns, as well as issues that were sub-acute or secondary at the time of the ED admission. This finding suggests the added value of the later follow-up, as it has the potential to support the increased identification of underlying or newly arising patient needs that may have gone unmet without a later follow-up. Later follow-up also presented a unique opportunity for improved transitions of care and care management relating to physician follow-up. The later time-point appears to facilitate scheduling of appointments that were recommended but had not yet been initiated, which was a pattern more commonly observed at this stage. The early follow-up proved critical for establishing initial connections to medical equipment, therapy, and home nursing services; however, later follow-up also added value where apparent 'missed connections' with services were concerned.

In examining the patient concerns and interventions directly from the telephone calls, our qualitative results show that there is a benefit to telephone follow-up after an emergency department visit. While Biese et al. found no benefit of a telephone call to older adults from the ED on readmission or death in primary outcomes, our results show that there are unmet needs after a hospital visit that benefit from phone follow-up and interventions [23]. The singular outcomes of readmission or death may not provide a complete picture as to the effects or benefits of a telephone follow-up after an ED visit. Hwang et al. encouraged expanding the scope of the outcomes assessed, beyond hospital admissions and ED revisits, as a necessary starting point for future work—including how ED interventions affect important outcomes such as perceived social support, use of home care services and physician referrals, and functional decline [24]. Our results show that during telephone follow-up after an ED visit, issues relating to older adult patients that can be eased by essential interventions, such as home services, medical equipment, social support, and physician referrals, can be initiated to improve quality of care.

4.2. Strengths and Limitations

The qualitative design of this study allowed for the identification of novel patterns and themes that elucidate the value of two distinct time-points for follow-ups with patients admitted to the emergency department. The comparison of themes between two time-points illustrated the distinct benefits of each stage of follow-up. The study is limited, however, in that the nature of these data and methods do not permit for parametric statistical analysis; therefore, the frequencies with which these themes arose in early and late follow-up, while informative descriptively, cannot be applied to establish the significance of the observed differences.

4.3. Recommendations and Future Directions

Follow-up phone calls following an emergency department visit, occurring at two time-points, identified the questions and unmet needs of older adult patients after emergency department discharge. The geriatrics nurse liaisons (GNLs) were able to remedy these concerns and needs, thus establishing the value of follow-up phone calls within the context of the GEDI program. These findings suggest that both short-term and longer-term follow-up telephone calls are critical, as they each promote the management of distinct problems by allowing the GNLs to identify needs that arise at different stages post-discharge.

A future focus for the investigation of GEDI follow-up will be establishing the impact of these telephone calls on quantitative, outcomes-based metrics, such as 30-day readmission. The readmission of older adults following emergency room discharge is a pressing issue for patients and hospitals, with rates of 30-day readmission estimated to reach between 12 and 20% [18,19]. Based on our findings, GEDI follow-up calls provide an opportunity to connect older adults with the care that they need and demonstrate concrete incidences of direct intervention taken by GNLs to promote patient access to medical care, as well as non-medical services. Important next steps in this line of research include demonstrating the downstream impacts of reaching patients in this way on outcome measures and using the newly identified themes to direct the improvement of discharge interventions, such as the GEDI program.

Author Contributions: All the authors made substantial contributions to the conception/design of the work. L.M.: Data analysis, preparation of the draft manuscript, and finalization of the manuscript. L.X.: Data analysis and preparation and finalization of the manuscript. S.D.: Concept, study design, and preparation and finalization of the manuscript. V.R.-Z.: Study design and preparation and finalization of the manuscript. L.A.L.: Concept, study design, data analysis, and preparation and finalization of the manuscript.

Funding: This research received no external funding.

Conflicts of Interest: The authors have neither current nor potential financial or personal conflicts of interest to report.

Impact Statement: We certify that this work is novel or confirmatory of recent novel clinical research. The potential impact of this research on clinical care or health policy includes the following: (1) Providing data supporting the use of follow-up phone calls in emergency department protocols for the care of older adults. (2) Identifying key care needs of older adults discharged from the emergency department that may be addressed through follow-up phone calls.

References

1. U.S. Census Bureau. The Population 65 Years and Older in the United States. Available online: https://www.census.gov/library/publications/2018/acs/acs-38.html (accessed on 5 December 2018).
2. Rui, P.; Kang, K. National Hospital Ambulatory Medical Care Survey: 2014 Emergency Department Summary Tables. HHS 2014. United States Department of Health and Human Services (Online). Available online: https://www.cdc.gov/nchs/data/nhamcs/web_tables/2014_ed_web_tables.pdf (accessed on 2 January 2018).
3. McCusker, J.; Cardin, S.; Bellavance, F.; Belzile, E. Return to the emergency department among elders: Patterns and predictors. *Acad. Emerg. Med.* **2000**, *7*, 249–259. [CrossRef] [PubMed]
4. Pines, J.M.; Mullins, P.M.; Cooper, J.K.; Feng, L.B.; Roth, K.E. National trends in emergency department use, care patterns, and quality of care of older adults in the United States. *J. Am. Geriatr. Soc.* **2013**, *61*, 12–17. [CrossRef] [PubMed]
5. Creditor, M.C. Hazards of hospitalization of the elderly. *Ann. Intern. Med.* **1993**, *118*, 219–223. [CrossRef] [PubMed]
6. Carpenter, C.R.; Bromley, M.; Caterino, J.M.; Chun, A.; Gerson, L.W.; Greenspan, J.; Hwang, U.; John, D.P.; Lyons, W.L.; Platts-Mills, T.F.; et al. Optimal older adult emergency care: Introducing multidisciplinary geriatric emergency department guidelines from the American College of Emergency Physicians, American Geriatrics Society, Emergency Nurses Association, and Society for Academic Emergency Medicine. *J. Am. Geriatr. Soc.* **2014**, *62*, 1360–1363. [PubMed]
7. McCusker, J.; Bellavance, F.; Cardin, S.; Trepanier, S.; Verdon, J.; Ardman, O. Detection of older people at increased risk of adverse health outcomes after an emergency visit: The ISAR screening tool. *J. Am. Geriatr. Soc.* **1999**, *47*, 1229–1237. [CrossRef] [PubMed]
8. Mion, L.C.; Palmer, R.M.; Anetzberger, G.J.; Meldon, S.W. Establishing a case-finding and referral system for at-risk older individuals in the emergency department setting: The SIGNET model. *J. Am. Geriatr. Soc.* **2001**, *49*, 1379–1386. [CrossRef] [PubMed]
9. Aldeen, A.Z.; Courtney, D.M.; Lindquist, L.A.; Dresden, S.M.; Gravenor, S.J.; GEDI-WISE Investigators. Geriatric emergency department innovations: Preliminary data for the geriatric nurse liaison model. *J. Am. Geriatr. Soc.* **2014**, *62*, 1781–1785. [CrossRef] [PubMed]
10. Hwang, U.; Rosenberg, M.S.; Dresden, S.M. Geriatrics Emergency Department—The GEDI WISE Program. In *Geriatrics Models of Care*; Springer: Berlin/Heidelberg, Germany, 2015; pp. 201–209.
11. Dudas, V.; Bookwalter, T.; Kerr, K.M.; Pagentilat, S.Z. The impact of follow-up telephone calls to patients after hospitalization. *Am. J. Med.* **2001**, *111*, 26–30. [CrossRef]
12. Harrison, J.D.; Auerbach, A.D.; Quinn, K.; Kynoch, E.; Mourad, M. Assessing the impact of nurse post-discharge telephone calls on 30-day hospital readmission rates. *J. Gen. Intern. Med.* **2014**, *29*, 1519–1525. [CrossRef] [PubMed]
13. Chande, V.T.; Exum, V. Follow-up phone calls after an emergency department visit. *Pediatrics* **1994**, *93*, 513–514. [PubMed]

14. Dockery, F.; Rajkumar, C.; Chapman, C.; Bulpitt, C.; Nicholl, C. The effect of reminder calls in reducing non-attendance rates at care of the elderly clinics. *Postgrad. Med. J.* **2001**, *77*, 37–39. [CrossRef] [PubMed]
15. Karam, G.; Radden, Z.; Berall, L.E.; Cheng, C.; Gruneir, A. Efficacy of emergency department-based interventions designed to reduce repeat visits and other adverse outcomes for older patients after discharge: A systematic review. *Geriatr. Gerontol. Int.* **2015**, *15*, 1107–1117. [CrossRef] [PubMed]
16. Nasreddine, Z.S.; Phillips, N.A.; Bédirian, V.; Charbonneau, S.; Whitehead, V.; Collin, I.; Cummings, J.L.; Chertkow, H. The Montreal Cognitive Assessment, MoCA: A brief screening tool for mild cognitive impairment. *J. Am. Geriatr. Soc.* **2005**, *53*, 695–699. [CrossRef] [PubMed]
17. Guba, E.G.; Lincoln, Y.S. Competing paradigms in qualitative research. *Handb. Qual. Res.* **1994**, *2*, 105.
18. Charmaz, K. Qualitative interviewing and grounded theory analysis. In *Handbook of Interview Research: Context and Method*; Gubrium, J.F., Holstein, J.A., Eds.; Sage: Thousand Oaks, CA, USA, 2011; pp. 675–694.
19. Morse, J.M. The significance of saturation. *Qual. Health Res.* **1995**, *5*, 147–149. [CrossRef]
20. Morse, J.M. Determining sample size. *Qual. Health Res.* **2000**, *10*, 3–5. [CrossRef]
21. Guest, G.; Bunce, A.; Johnson, L. How many interviews are enough? An experiment with data saturation and variability. *Field Methods* **2006**, *18*, 59–82. [CrossRef]
22. Crouch, M.; McKenzie, H. The logic of small samples in interview based qualitative research. *Soc. Sci. Inf.* **2006**, *45*, 483–499. [CrossRef]
23. Biese, K.; Busby-Whitehead, J.; Cai, J.; Stearns, S.C.; Roberts, E.; Mihas, P.; Emmett, D.; Zhou, Q.; Farmer, F.; Kizer, J.S. Telephone follow-up for older adults discharged to home from the emergency department: A pragmatic randomized controlled trial. *J. Am. Geriatr. Soc.* **2018**, *66*, 452–458. [CrossRef] [PubMed]
24. Ula Hwang, S. Nicole Hastings and Katherine Ramos, Improving Emergency Department Discharge Care with Telephone Follow-Up. Does It Connect? *J. Am. Geriatr. Soc.* **2017**, *66*, 436–438. [CrossRef] [PubMed]

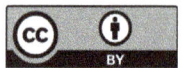

© 2019 by the authors. Licensee MDPI, Basel, Switzerland. This article is an open access article distributed under the terms and conditions of the Creative Commons Attribution (CC BY) license (http://creativecommons.org/licenses/by/4.0/).

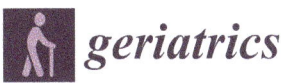

Article

Comprehensive Geriatric Assessment and Nutrition-Related Assessment: A Cross-Sectional Survey for Health Professionals

Junko Ueshima [1,*], Keisuke Maeda [2], Hidetaka Wakabayashi [3], Shinta Nishioka [4], Saori Nakahara [5] and Yoji Kokura [6]

1. Department of Clinical Nutrition and Food Service, NTT Medical Center Tokyo, Tokyo 141-0022, Japan
2. Palliative Care Center, Aichi Medical University, Aichi 480-1195, Japan; kskmaeda@aichi-med-u.ac.jp
3. Department of Rehabilitation Medicine, Yokohama City University Medical Center, Yokohama 232-0024, Japan; noventurenoglory@gmail.com
4. Department of Clinical Nutrition and Food Services, Nagasaki Rehabilitation Hospital, Nagasaki 850-0854, Japan; shintacks@yahoo.co.jp
5. Department of Nutrition, Suzuka General Hospital, Suzuka 513-8630, Japan; mikuhiroto1210@gmail.com
6. Department of Clinical Nutrition, Keiju Medical Center, Nanao 926-8605, Japan; yojikokura@hotmail.com
* Correspondence: j.ueshima@gmail.com; Tel.: +81-3-3448-6111

Received: 26 December 2018; Accepted: 12 February 2019; Published: 15 February 2019

Abstract: (1) Background: It is important to assess physical and nutritional status using the Comprehensive Geriatric Assessment (CGA). However, the correlation between the CGA usage and nutritional-related assessments remain unclear. This study aims to clarify the correlation between the CGA usage and other nutritional-related assessments. (2) Methods: We conducted a questionnaire survey on clinical use of CGA, assessment of sarcopenia/sarcopenic dysphagia/cachexia, and defining nutritional goals/the Nutrition Care Process/the International Classification of Functioning, Disability, and Health (ICF)/the Kuchi–Kara Taberu Index. (3) Results: The number of respondents was 652 (response rate, 12.0%), including 77 who used the CGA in the general practice. The univariate analyses revealed that participants using the CGA tended to assess sarcopenia ($P = 0.029$), sarcopenic dysphagia ($P = 0.001$), and define nutritional goals ($P < 0.001$). Multivariate logistic regression analyses for the CGA usage revealed that using ICF ($P < 0.001$), assessing sarcopenia ($P = 0.001$), sarcopenic dysphagia ($P = 0.022$), and cachexia ($P = 0.039$), and defining nutritional goals ($P = 0.001$) were statistically significant after adjusting for confounders. (4) Conclusions: There are correlations between the use of CGA and evaluation of sarcopenia, sarcopenic dysphagia, and cachexia and nutritional goals.

Keywords: comprehensive geriatric assessment; multicomponent assessment; rehabilitation nutrition; sarcopenia; sarcopenic dysphagia

1. Introduction

The rapidly aging society warrants continuous advancements of the conventional medical care [1,2]. As frail older adults should have access to comprehensive medical and nursing care, provision of comprehensive care using multicomponent assessment is imperative [2]. The Comprehensive Geriatric Assessment (CGA) is a multidimensional, interdisciplinary diagnostic and treatment process that is designed to collect data about medical aspects of frail older adults [3,4]. The primary components of various models of the CGA comprise the coordinated multidisciplinary assessment, geriatric medicine expertise, determining medical, physical, social, and psychological problems, and the creation of a care plan involving appropriate rehabilitation [4]. Compared to typical medical care, the CGA implementation enhances the survival time of older adults, increases the duration during which they can live at home, and, perhaps, improves cognitive functions [1,4], improving their quality of life (QOL). Despite being recommended to be used in in the clinical practice, the CGA remains only partially utilized [5].

Sarcopenia, a key contributor of frailty [6], is a syndrome characterized by the presence of both the muscle mass and muscle function reduction due to aging, inactivity, malnutrition, and conditions such as cachexia [7]. Reportedly, sarcopenia is associated with an increased mortality and healthcare costs and declined QOL [8], and is considered as a severe public health-related concern [8,9]. Recently, some studies have described sarcopenic dysphagia (dysphagia due to sarcopenia in the whole body and swallowing-related muscles.) [10–14], which is occasionally detected in older adults and is related to physical deterioration, inadequate nutrition management, and cognitive decline [15]. Perhaps multicomponent assessment, such as the assessment of physical, social, and psychological problems, appropriate rehabilitation, and nutrition management could be necessary for the treatment [14,15], necessitating the early diagnosis of sarcopenia. In Nakahara et al. [16], we clarified the evaluation of sarcopenia and cachexia among different occupations, but when these items were evaluated remains unclear. In the rapidly aging society of Japan, the number of older adults with sarcopenia, nutritional deficiency, weakness, and disability are increasing at an alarming rate [17]. Therefore, it is important to assess physical functions and nutritional status as well as using CGA and to extract patients at risk early.

The usage of the multicomponent assessment is desirable to evaluate the elderly clinically and has been projected to attain a shared understanding of assessment and intervention goals. Besides the CGA, there are other multicomponent tools that clinically assess older adults such as the International Classification of Functioning, Disability, and Health (ICF) and the Kuchi–Kara Taberu Index (KT index) [18]. Wakabayashi et al. [11] advocates care that can maximize the physical function, physical activity, and social participation by assessing patients by ICF, including the nutritional status. Maeda et al. [18] recommended the multicomponent assessment and nutrition management for patients with eating and swallowing problems using the KT index. Recently, ICF-Dietetics [19] has been established as a systematically problem-solving method for ICF-related nutritional issues. The CGA usage mandates defining nutritional goals and controlling nutrition using nutritional problem-solving methods, such as the Nutrition Care Process (NCP) [20] and nutrition management, with a common understanding among healthcare workers in different occupations. Based on these, Wakabayashi [17] suggested providing high-quality nutritional care using the rehabilitation nutrition care process to people with disability and frailty. The rehabilitation nutrition care process assesses frailty, sarcopenia, dysphagia, and cachexia after using multicomponent assessment tools such as ICF or CGA and KT index. However, the rehabilitation nutrition care process has just begun, and the correlation between the CGA usage and the assessment of sarcopenia, cachexia, and sarcopenic dysphagia and defining nutritional goals using the NCP remain unclear. Moreover, the correlation between the CGA usage and the ICF usage and the KT index remains unknown.

In addition, a medical fee has been obtained since 2008 owing to the implementation of the CGA in Japan. Kihon Checklist [21] is an example of the CGA; although the assessment of frailty and assessment of muscle strength and physical functions are included in its components, the assessment of muscle mass and cachexia is not included.

Therefore, this study aims to elucidate the implementation rate and correlation between using the CGA and using nutrition-related assessment items, such as assessment of sarcopenia, cachexia, and sarcopenic dysphagia, NCP, defining nutritional goals, through a questionnaire-based survey. It also explains the implementation rate of CGA among different types of healthcare professionals and settings. Furthermore, this study intends to assess the correlation between the CGA usage and the use of other multicomponent tools, including the ICF and KT index.

2. Materials and Methods

2.1. Study Design and Setting

Between December 9, 2016, and January 16, 2017, we conducted a cross-sectional study using questionnaires. The questionnaire respondents were members of the Japanese Association of Rehabilitation Nutrition, which was established in 2011 and includes 5520 members from various medical and healthcare specialties. We conducted the survey online and anonymously to protect respondents' personal information and guarantee confidentiality.

2.2. Ethical Considerations

This study was performed following the ethical guidelines of the Declaration of Helsinki and was approved by the Ethics Committee of Suzuka General Hospital at Mie prefecture in Japan (No. 161). With answers to the questionnaire, we explained to the participants that they consented to the research and were given responses. For the protection of personal information in completed questionnaires, full confidentiality was given to respondents' data.

2.3. Participants

In this study, we enrolled respondents who provided consent to participate in the survey and responded to the questionnaire. Of note, those with missing data or duplications were excluded from the analysis.

2.4. Data Collection

We conducted the survey online, and it took approximately 5 min to complete the online questionnaire that comprised selective questions with dichotomous choice (yes/no). The consistency of the questionnaire content was evaluated by researchers. After several investigators conducted preliminary tests, the questionnaire content was enhanced regarding phrases, forms, length, consistency, and ease of answering, followed by converting into an actual survey. Table A1 lists the questions asked in the survey.

2.5. Parameters

In this study, we assessed parameters such as the standard implementation of the CGA, ICF, KT index, sarcopenia, sarcopenic dysphagia, cachexia, defining nutritional intervention goals, and the usage of NCP. The characterization of each evaluation item is in the Appendix (Table A2).

2.6. Statistical Analysis

Data analysis was performed on a sample size of >664 respondents, under the assumption of two-choice questions, and 50% selection with a 5% error based on 99% reliability. We expressed all categorical variables as the number of individuals and percentages. In addition, we performed a comparison of groups using the χ^2 test.

All quantitative variables were expressed as median (interquartile ranges). We used the Mann–Whitney U-test to compare values of the length of work experience. In addition, univariate and multivariate logistic regression analyses were performed to estimate the adjusted odds ratios (OR). Of note, the confounders were occupations, affiliations, and length of work experience. We performed all statistical procedures using EZR [22] software version 1.31, which was developed from the open-source statistical software R [23]. Furthermore, we considered $P < 0.05$ as statistically significant.

3. Results

Of 660 respondents, we excluded 8 (1.2%) from analyses because of incomprehensible answers. Consequently, the number of valid respondents was 652 (response rate, 12.0%). Table 1 summarizes the characteristics of the study cohort. The leading occupation of respondents was registered dietitian (28.2%), followed by a physical therapist (26.4%) and speech therapist (15.5%). Affiliations were with acute care (37.9%), convalescent rehabilitation (26.5%), nursing homes (10.4%), home care service (10.3%), long-term care (6.9%), and others (8%). Besides, the median work experience was 12 (range, 7–18) years.

Overall, 77 (11.8%) respondents were using the CGA in the general practice. The univariate analysis revealed that people using the CGA were more likely to assess sarcopenia ($P = 0.029$), sarcopenic dysphagia ($P = 0.001$), and define nutritional goals ($P < 0.001$). In contrast, using the ICF ($P = 0.051$), KT index ($P = 0.120$), and NCP ($P = 0.144$) and assessing cachexia ($P = 0.054$) was not significantly different (see Table 2).

The logistic regression analyses established a correlation between the CGA usage and several factors (see Table 3); these factors included using the ICF (adjusted OR, 3.01; 95% confidence interval [CI]: 1.63–3.57; $P < 0.001$), assessing sarcopenia (adjusted OR, 2.60; 95% CI: 1.50–4.50; $P = 0.001$), assessing sarcopenic dysphagia (adjusted OR, 1.86; 95% CI: 1.09–3.16; $P = 0.022$), assessing cachexia (adjusted OR, 1.86; 95% CI: 1.03–3.34; $P = 0.039$), and setting nutritional goals (adjusted OR, 2.79; 95% CI: 1.56–4.98; $P = 0.001$), which we observed with a statistical significance. Furthermore, the use of the KT index and NCP did not correlate with the CGA use.

Table 1. Demographic Characteristics of Participants.

Characteristics, n (%)	All	Usage of Comprehensive Geriatric Assessment		P-Value
		No	Yes	
Total Occupation	652 (100)	575 (88.2)	77 (11.8)	
Registered dietitian	184 (28.2)	162 (88.0)	22 (12.0)	0.01 [a]
Physical therapist	172 (26.4)	156 (90.7)	16 (9.3)	
Speech therapist	101 (15.5)	93 (92.1)	8 (7.9)	
Nurse	60 (9.2)	54 (90.0)	6 (10.0)	
Medical doctor	43 (6.6)	32 (74.4)	11 (25.6)	
Occupational therapist	36 (5.5)	33 (91.7)	3 (8.3)	
Dental hygienist	24 (3.7)	22 (91.7)	2 (8.3)	
Dentist	24 (3.7)	18 (75.0)	6 (25.0)	
Pharmacist	7 (1.1)	4 (57.1)	3 (42.9)	
Certified care worker	1 (0.1)	1 (100.0)	0 (0.0)	
Affiliation				
Acute care	247 (37.9)	231 (40.2)	16 (20.8)	0.02 [a]
Convalescent rehabilitation	173 (26.5)	149 (25.9)	24 (31.2)	
Nursing home	68 (10.4)	59 (10.3)	9 (11.7)	
Homecare service	67 (10.3)	53 (9.2)	14 (18.2)	
Medical care or long-term care	45 (6.9)	39 (6.8)	6 (7.8)	
Others	52 (8.0)	44 (7.7)	8 (10.4)	
Work experience				
Year(s), median (25–75%)	12 (7–18)	12 (7–18)	11 (7–20)	0.85 [b]

[a] Chi-square test; [b] Mann–Whitney U-test.

Table 2. Univariate Analysis of Factors Associated with Usage of Comprehensive Geriatric Assessment.

Factor, n (%)	All	Usage of Comprehensive Geriatric Assessment		P-Value
		No	Yes	
Using the ICF				
No	289 (44.3)	263 (45.7)	26 (33.8)	0.05
Yes	363 (55.7)	312 (54.3)	51 (66.2)	
Using the KT index				
No	557 (85.4)	496 (86.3)	61 (79.2)	0.12
Yes	95 (14.6)	79 (13.7)	16 (20.8)	
Assessing sarcopenia				
No	315 (48.3)	287 (49.9)	28 (36.4)	0.03
Yes	337 (51.7)	288 (50.1)	49 (63.6)	
Assessing sarcopenic dysphagia				
No	432 (66.3)	394 (68.5)	38 (49.4)	0.001
Yes	220 (33.7)	181 (31.5)	39 (50.6)	
Assessing cachexia				
No	478 (73.3)	429 (74.6)	49 (63.6)	0.05
Yes	174 (26.7)	146 (25.4)	28 (36.4)	
Setting nutritional goal				
No	359 (55.1)	333 (57.9)	26 (33.8)	<0.001
Yes	293 (44.9)	242 (42.1)	51 (66.2)	
Using Nutrition Care Process				
No	569 (87.3)	506 (88.0)	63 (81.8)	0.14
Yes	83 (12.7)	69 (12.0)	14 (18.2)	

Abbreviations: ICF, International Classification of Functioning, Disability and Health; KT index, Kuchi–Kara Taberu Index.

Table 3. Odds Ratio of Comprehensive Geriatric Assessment Usage in Uni- and Multi-Variate Logistic Regression Analyses.

Dependent Variables	Usage of Comprehensive Geriatric Assessment					
	Unadjusted OR	95% CI	P-Value	Adjusted OR	95% CI	P-Value
Using the ICF	1.65	0.98–2.84	0.05	3.01	1.63–5.57	<0.001
Using the KT index	1.66	0.84–3.07	0.12	1.76	0.91–3.43	0.10
Assessing sarcopenia	1.74	1.04–2.97	0.03	2.60	1.50–4.50	0.02
Assessing sarcopenic dysphagia	2.23	1.34–3.72	0.001	1.86	1.09–3.16	0.001
Assessing cachexia	1.68	0.98–2.84	0.05	1.86	1.03–3.34	0.04
Setting nutritional goal	2.70	1.60–4.64	<0.001	2.79	1.56–4.98	0.001
Using Nutrition Care Process	1.63	0.80–3.14	0.14	1.59	0.75–3.37	0.23

For each multivariate regression model, usage of CGA was adjusted by occupations, affiliations, and length of work experience. Abbreviations: ICF, International Classification of Functioning, Disability and Health; KT index, Kuchi–Kara Taberu Index; OR, odds ratio; 95% CI, 95% confidence interval.

4. Discussion

In brief, this study revealed three significant findings. First, it was suggested that participants using the CGA may have assessed sarcopenia or sarcopenic dysphagia more frequently in the daily clinical practice than those not using the CGA. Second, participants using the CGA defined nutritional goals more frequently; however, no significant difference was observed in using the NCP. Third, the percentage of people using the CGA was as low as 11.8%.

Participants using the CGA may have assessed sarcopenia or sarcopenic dysphagia more frequently in the daily clinical practice than those not using the CGA. Although there have been few studies on the relevance of assessing the CGA and sarcopenia. In recent studies, assessment of frailty was included as a component of CGA, but there was no sarcopenia [24]. Kihon Checklist [21] is a sample implementation of the CGA in Japan. It includes assessment of frailty, muscle strength, and physical functions in its components, and it has one aspect that motivates the assessment of sarcopenia. Sarcopenia is not only related to the physical activity and dysfunction [25,26] but also with several other factors, including independence [27,28] and cognitive function [29] of the daily life. In addition, sarcopenic dysphagia correlates with nutrition, activity (physical activity and swallowing), and cognitive function, which are causal factors of secondary sarcopenia [15]. Reportedly, the prevalence of sarcopenia among older adults is 1–29% in community dwellers, 14–33% in long-term care facilities, and 10–35% in acute-care hospitals [30,31]. Furthermore, it is a factor that predicts the life expectancy and disability. In fact, it is imperative to screen older adults who are susceptible to sarcopenia and sarcopenic dysphagia in the CGA and intervene at an early stage. As the CGA is the accepted gold standard for caring for frail older people in hospitals [24], it is essential to assess sarcopenia and sarcopenic dysphagia as a prolongation of the nutritional assessment and physical function evaluation of the CGA.

Participants using the CGA define nutritional goals more frequently; however, we observed no statistically significant difference in using the NCP. DiMaria-Ghalili et al. [32] reported that because all regions of the CGA and nutritional status were related, the nutritional assessment in the CGA facilitated the early recognition of nutritional risk factors or malnutrition, raising the possibility of a timely intervention. A study reported that it is crucial to illustrate the setting of nutritional goals at the time of the intervention after the nutrition assessment [33]. Although defining nutrition goals is encouraged for the NCP, a method of systematically solving nutrition-related problems, we observed no significant differences in using the NCP. Perhaps, participants related the nutritional assessment to the CGA, but the nutrition goal setting was implemented by methods other than the NCP. In Japan, NCP education has been initiated only recently for registered dietitians, and the NCP has not yet been applied in several occupations. In future, it will be crucial to define nutritional goals using nutrition-related problem-solving methods that could be shared among multiple occupations in Japan.

Among our study participants, the implementation rate of the CGA was as low as 11.8%, which was particularly low in acute-care hospitals. Apparently, the interdisciplinary work is necessary for the CGA implementation. We conjecture that the emergency departments of acute-care hospitals prioritize professional care over the CGA [5], or such an interdisciplinary working model has not been established [34]. Gladman et al. [5] reported that the CGA is challenging to comprehend and implement, even among those who care for the elderly. Li et al. [34] reported that even when the CGA was indicated, its implementation rate was as low as 20% because of inadequate education. In Japan, CGA education exists for medical doctors and dentists provided by gerontologists, but such an education is not provided for other medical professionals, although it is essential that all healthcare professionals should have access to adequate education. We need to clarify the reason why we are assessing sarcopenia and not using CGA, although we could not describe in this research. Thereby, we believe that the issue at the clinical practice will be highlighted.

This study has several limitations. First, based on the questionnaire response rate of only 12.0%, it is difficult to generalize our findings to the entire country. Second, it remains unclear how the questionnaire respondents diagnosed sarcopenia, sarcopenic dysphagia, and cachexia. When conducting similar research next time, it is necessary to describe diagnostic criteria of sarcopenia, sarcopenic dysphagia, and cachexia. If we clarify the reason why participants assess sarcopenia, sarcopenic dysphagia, cachexia, and the CGA, we can get more insights for clinical practice.

5. Conclusions

In conclusion, this study establishes correlations between the CGA usage and evaluation of sarcopenia, sarcopenic dysphagia, and cachexia and nutritional goals. In addition, those using the CGA are highly likely to assess older adults with a more multidimensional approach. However, the presence of few implementers is problematic. It is essential to extract older adults susceptible to sarcopenia at an early stage with an appropriate care plan, including the rehabilitation and nutrition management. Therefore, in the future it will be necessary to include items for the evaluation of sarcopenia, sarcopenic dysphagia, and cachexia in the CGA.

Author Contributions: J.U., concept and design, data acquisition, data interpretation, drafting the manuscript; K.M., H.W., S.N. (Shinta Nishioka), S.N. (Saori Nakahara), and Y.K., concept and design, data interpretation, critical revision of the manuscript. All the authors revised the manuscript critically for important intellectual content and approved the final version of the manuscript.

Funding: The authors have no funding or support disclosure.

Conflicts of Interest: The authors have no conflicts of interest.

Appendix A

Table A1. Questionnaire contents.

Questions	Options
Q1. What is your occupation?	Registered dietitian Physical therapist Speech therapist Nurse Medical doctor Occupational therapist Dental hygienist Dentist Pharmacist Certified Care Worker
Q2. What is your sex?	Male Female
Q3. What is your affiliation?	Acute care Recovery rehabilitation Long-term care health facility Homecare service Medical care or long-term care Others
Q4. How long is your work experience?	
Q5. Do you use the CGA?	Yes/No
Q6. Do you assess sarcopenia?	Yes/No
Q7. Do you assess sarcopenic dysphagia?	Yes/No
Q8. Do you assess cachexia?	Yes/No
Q9. Do you set nutritional goals?	Yes/No
Q10. Do you use KT index?	Yes/No
Q11. Do you use the Nutrition Care Process?	Yes/No
Q12. Do you use the ICF?	Yes/No

Abbreviations: CGA, Comprehensive geriatric assessment; KT index, Kuchi–Kara Taberu Index; ICF, International Classification of Functioning, Disability and Health.

Table A2. The characterization of each evaluation items.

The ICF	The WHO framework for measuring health and disability at both individual and population levels. It is classified according to a combination of alphabet and number, and it consists of three factors, "physical and mental function/physical structure," "activity" and "participation," and influential factors, such as "environment" and "individual" [35].
The KT index	A simplified, validated tool that comprehensively assesses and intervenes in problems associated with eating and swallowing. The index comprises the following 13 items: (1) willingness to eat, (2) overall condition, (3) respiratory condition, (4) oral condition, (5) cognitive function while eating, (6) oral preparatory and propulsive phases, (7) severity of pharyngeal dysphagia, (8) position and endurance while eating, (9) eating behavior, (10) daily living activities, (11) food intake level, (12) food modification, and (13) nutritional status [18]. As each item is rated from 1 (worst) to 5 (best) points, the KT index ranges from 13 to 65 and is drawn with a radar chart that facilitates determining strong and weak items to ascertain items that caregivers need to emphasize and recognize the effect of an intervention by comparing before and after results.
The NCP	A systematic approach to provide high-quality nutritional care to patients/clients and is the unique function of nutrition in a standardized language through four related steps as follows: (1) nutrition assessment, (2) nutrition diagnosis, (3) nutrition management, and (4) nutrition monitoring and evaluation [20].

Abbreviations: WHO, World Health Organization; KT index, Kuchi–Kara Taberu Index; ICF, International Classification of Functioning, Disability and Health; NCP, Nutrition Care Process.

References

1. Ellis, G.; Whitehead, M.A.; Robinson, D.; O'Neill, D.; Langhorne, P. Comprehensive geriatric assessment for older adults admitted to hospital: Meta-analysis of randomized controlled trials. *BMJ* **2011**, *27*, 343. [CrossRef] [PubMed]
2. Arai, H.; Ouchi, Y.; Toba, K.; Endo, T.; Shimokado, K.; Tsubota, K.; Matsuo, S.; Mori, H.; Yumura, W.; Yokode, M.; et al. Japan as the front-runner of super-aged societies: Perspectives from medicine and medical care in Japan. *Geriatr. Gerontol. Int.* **2015**, *15*, 673–687. [CrossRef] [PubMed]
3. Rubenstein, L.Z.; Siu, A.L.; Wieland, D. Comprehensive geriatric assessment: Toward understanding its efficacy. *Aging* **1989**, *1*, 87–98. [CrossRef]
4. Ellis, G.; Whitehead, M.A.; O'Neill, D.; Langhorne, P.; Robinson, D. Comprehensive geriatric assessment for older adults admitted to hospital. *Cochrane Database Syst. Rev.* **2011**. [CrossRef]
5. Gladman, J.R.; Conroy, S.P.A.; Ranhoff, H.; Gordon, A.L. New horizons in the implementation and research of comprehensive geriatric assessment: Knowing, doing and the 'know-do' gap. *Age Ageing* **2016**, *45*, 194–200. [CrossRef]
6. Fried, L.P.; Tangen, C.M.; Walston, J.; Newman, A.B.; Hirsch, C.; Gottdiener, J.; Seeman, T.; Tracy, R.; Kop, W.J.; Burke, G.; et al. Frailty in older adults: Evidence for a phenotype. *J. Gerontol. A Biol. Sci. Med. Sci.* **2001**, *56*, M146–M156. [CrossRef]
7. Cruz-Jentoft, A.J.; Baeyens, J.P.; Bauer, J.M.; Boirie, Y.; Cederholm, T.; Landi, F.; Martin, F.C.; Michel, J.P.; Rolland, Y.; Schneider, S.M.; et al. Sarcopenia: European consensus on definition and diagnosis: Report of the European Working Group on Sarcopenia in Older People. *Age Ageing* **2010**, *39*, 412–423. [CrossRef]
8. Beaudart, C.; Rizzoli, R.; Bruyère, O.; Reginster, J.Y.; Biver, E. Sarcopenia: Burden and challenges for public health. *Arch. Public Health* **2014**, *72*, 45. [CrossRef]
9. Bruyère, O.; Beaudart, C.; Locquet, M.; Buckinx, F.; Petermans, J.; Reginster, J.-Y. Sarcopenia as a public health problem. *Eur. Geriatr. Med.* **2016**, *7*, 272–275. [CrossRef]
10. Fujishima, I.; Fujiu-Kurachi, M.; Arai, H.; Hyodo, M.; Kagaya, H.; Maeda, K.; Mori, T.; Nishioka, S.; Oshima, F.; Ogawa, S.; et al. Sarcopenia and dysphagia: Position paper by four professional organizations. *Geriatr. Gerontol. Int.* **2019**, *19*. [CrossRef]
11. Wakabayashi, H.; Sakuma, K. Rehabilitation nutrition for sarcopenia with disability: A combination of both rehabilitation and nutrition care management. *J. Cachexia Sarcopenia Muscle* **2014**, *5*, 269–277. [CrossRef] [PubMed]
12. Kuroda, Y.; Kuroda, R. Relationship between thinness and swallowing function in Japanese older adults: Implications for sarcopenic dysphagia. *J. Am. Geriatr. Soc.* **2012**, *60*, 1785–1786. [CrossRef]
13. Maeda, K.; Akagi, J. Sarcopenia is an independent risk factor of dysphagia in hospitalized older people. *Geriatr. Gerontol. Int.* **2016**, *16*, 515–521. [CrossRef] [PubMed]
14. Wakabayashi, H. Presbyphagia and sarcopenic dysphagia: Association between aging, sarcopenia, and deglutition disorders. *J. Frailty Aging* **2014**, *3*, 97–103.
15. Maeda, K.; Takaki, M.; Akagi, J. Decreased skeletal muscle mass and risk factors of sarcopenic dysphagia: A prospective observational cohort study. *J. Gerontol. A Biol. Sci. Med. Sci* **2017**, *72*, 1290–1294. [CrossRef] [PubMed]
16. Saori, N.; Hidetaka, W.; Keisuke, M.; Shinta, N.; Yoji, K. Sarcopenia and cachexia evaluation in different healthcare settings: A questionnaire survey of health professionals. *Asia Pac. J. Clin. Nutr.* **2018**, *27*, 167–175.
17. Wakabayashi, H. Rehabilitation nutrition in general and family medicine. *J. Gen. Fam. Med.* **2017**, *18*, 153–154. [CrossRef]
18. Maeda, K.; Shamoto, H.; Wakabayashi, H.; Enomoto, J.; Takeichi, M.; Koyama, T. Reliability and validity of a simplified comprehensive assessment tool for feeding support: Kuchi-KaraTaberu Index. *J. Am. Geriatr. Soc.* **2016**, *64*, e248–e252. [CrossRef]
19. Gäbler, G.; Coenen, M.C.; Bolleurs, C.; Visser, W.K.; Runia, S.; Heerkens, Y.F.; Stamm, T.A. Toward harmonization of the Nutrition Care Process terminology and the International Classification of Functioning, Disability and Health-Dietetics: Results of a mapping exercise and implications for nutrition and dietetics practice and research. *J. Acad. Nutr. Diet.* **2018**, *118*, 13–20. [CrossRef]
20. Writing Group of the Nutrition Care Process/Standardized Language Committee. Nutrition Care Process and Model Part I: The 2008 Update. *J. Am. Diet. Assoc.* **2008**, *108*, 1113–1117. [CrossRef]

21. Sewo Sampaio, P.Y.; Sampaio, R.A.; Yamada, M.; Arai, H. Systematic review of the Kihon Checklist: Is it a reliable assessment of frailty? *Geriatr. Gerontol. Int.* **2016**, *16*, 893–902. [CrossRef] [PubMed]
22. Kanda, Y. Investigation of the freely available easy-to-use software 'EZR' for medical statistics. *Bone Marrow Transpl.* **2013**, *48*, 452–458. [CrossRef] [PubMed]
23. Institute for Statistics and Mathematics of Wirtschaftsuniversität Wien. The Comprehensive R Archive Network. 2009. Available online: https://cran.r-project.org/ (accessed on 8 March 2017).
24. Parker, S.G.; McCue, P.; Phelps, K.; McCleod, A.; Arora, S.; Nockels, K.; Kennedy, S.; Roberts, H.; Conroy, S. What is Comprehensive Geriatric Assessment (CGA)? An umbrella review. *Age Ageing* **2018**, *47*, 149–155. [CrossRef] [PubMed]
25. Tanimoto, Y.; Watanabe, M.; Sun, W.; Sugiura, Y.; Tsuda, Y.; Kimura, M.; Hayashida, I.; Kusabiraki, T.; Kono, K. Association between sarcopenia and higher-level functional capacity in daily living in community-dwelling elderly subjects in Japan. *Arch. Gerontol. Geriatr.* **2012**, *55*, e9–e13. [CrossRef] [PubMed]
26. Guralnik, J.M.; Ferrucci, L.; Pieper, C.F.; Leveille, S.G.; Markides, K.S.; Ostir, G.V.; Studenski, S.; Berkman, L.F.; Wallace, R.B. Lower extremity function and subsequent disability: Consistency across studies, predictive models, and value of gait speed alone compared with the short physical performance battery. *J. Gerontol. A Biol. Sci. Med. Sci.* **2000**, *55*, M221–M231. [CrossRef]
27. Maeda, K.; Shamoto, H.; Wakabayashi, H.; Akagi, J. Sarcopenia is highly prevalent in older medical patients with mobility limitation. *Nutr. Clin. Pr.* **2017**, *32*, 110–115. [CrossRef]
28. Janssen, I.; Baumgartner, R.N.; Ross, R.; Rosenberg, I.H.; Roubenoff, R. Skeletal muscle cutpoints associated with elevated physical disability risk in older men and women. *Am. J. Epidemiol.* **2004**, *159*, 413–421. [CrossRef] [PubMed]
29. Maeda, K.; Akagi, J. Cognitive impairment is independently associated with definitive and possible sarcopenia in hospitalized older adults: The prevalence and impact of comorbidities. *Geriatr. Gerontol. Int.* **2017**, *17*, 1048–1056. [CrossRef]
30. Bianchi, L.; Abete, P.; Bellelli, G.; Bo, M.; Cherubini, A.; Corica, F.; Di Bari, M.; Maggio, M.; Manca, G.M.; Rizzo, M.R.; et al. Prevalence and clinical correlates of sarcopenia, identified according to the EWGSOP definition and diagnostic algorithm, in hospitalized older people: The GLISTEN Study. *J. Gerontol. A Biol. Sci. Med. Sci.* **2017**, *72*, 1575–1581. [CrossRef]
31. Cruz-Jentoft, A.J.; Landi, F.; Schneider, S.M.; Zúñiga, C.; Arai, H.; Boirie, Y.; Chen, L.K.; Fielding, R.A.; Martin, F.C.; Michel, J.P.; et al. Prevalence of and interventions for sarcopenia in ageing adults: A systematic review. Report of the International Sarcopenia Initiative (EWGSOP and IWGS). *Age Ageing* **2014**, *43*, 748–759. [CrossRef]
32. DiMaria-Ghalili, R.A. Integrating nutrition in the Comprehensive Geriatric Assessment. *Nutr. Clin. Pr.* **2014**, *29*, 420–427. [CrossRef] [PubMed]
33. Cederholm, T.; Barazzoni, R.; Austin, P.; Ballmer, P.; Biolo, G.; Bischoff, S.C.; Compher, C.; Correia, I.; Higashiguchi, T.; Holst, M.; et al. ESPEN guidelines on definitions and terminology of clinical nutrition. *Clin. Nutr.* **2017**, *36*, 49–64. [CrossRef] [PubMed]
34. Li, Y.; Wang, S.; Wang, L.X.; Meng, Z.M.; Li, J.; Dong, B.R. Is comprehensive geriatric assessment recognized and applied in Southwest China? A survey from Sichuan Association of Geriatrics. *J. Am. Med. Dir. Assoc.* **2013**, *14*, 775.e1–775.e3. [CrossRef] [PubMed]
35. World Health Organization. Available online: http://www.who.int/classifications/icf/en/ (accessed on 11 January 2019).

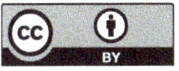

© 2019 by the authors. Licensee MDPI, Basel, Switzerland. This article is an open access article distributed under the terms and conditions of the Creative Commons Attribution (CC BY) license (http://creativecommons.org/licenses/by/4.0/).

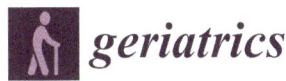

Review

Comprehensive Geriatric Assessment as a Versatile Tool to Enhance the Care of the Older Person Diagnosed with Cancer

Janine Overcash [1,*], Nikki Ford [2], Elizabeth Kress [2], Caitlin Ubbing [2] and Nicole Williams [2]

1. The College of Nursing, The Ohio State University, 1585 Neil Ave, Newton Hall, Columbus, OH 43201, USA
2. Stephanie Spielman Comprehensive Breast Center, The Ohio State University, 1145 Olentangy River Road, Columbus, OH 43121, USA; Nikki.Ford@osumc.edu (N.F.); Eizabeth.Kress@osumc.edu (E.K.); Caitlin.Ubbing@osumc.edu (C.U.); Nicole.Williams@osumc.edu (N.W.)
* Correspondence: Overcash.1@osu.edu

Received: 20 May 2019; Accepted: 20 June 2019; Published: 24 June 2019

Abstract: The comprehensive geriatric assessment (CGA) is a versatile tool for the care of the older person diagnosed with cancer. The purpose of this article is to detail how a CGA can be tailored to Ambulatory Geriatric Oncology Programs (AGOPs) in academic cancer centers and to community oncology practices with varying levels of resources. The Society for International Oncology in Geriatrics (SIOG) recommends CGA as a foundation for treatment planning and decision-making for the older person receiving care for a malignancy. A CGA is often administered by a multidisciplinary team (MDT) composed of professionals who provide geriatric-focused cancer care. CGA can be used as a one-time consult for surgery, chemotherapy, or radiation therapy providers to predict treatment tolerance or as an ongoing part of patient care to manage malignant and non-malignant issues. Administrative support and proactive infrastructure planning to address scheduling, referrals, and provider communication are critical to the effectiveness of the CGA.

Keywords: comprehensive geriatric assessment; CGA; multidisciplinary team; senior adult; cancer

---

Caring for the older adult who is diagnosed with cancer can be a complex orchestration of managing existing comorbid conditions, cancer care, caregiver concerns, while maintaining quality of life [1–4]. Older people have unique healthcare needs compared to younger adults who may not have challenges regarding comorbidities [4–7], functional ability [8], transportation and social support [9]. Many academic and community cancer centers establish some type of multidisciplinary geriatric oncology program to meet the needs of the older person [10–15]. The central element associated with a geriatric oncology program is a comprehensive geriatric assessment (CGA). Despite the evidence showing the benefits of CGA, only 9% and 8% of Phase II and Phase III clinical trials use CGA [16]. Many healthcare settings do not use CGA also because of time constraints, availability of a multidisciplinary team, and lack of professionals trained in geriatrics/gerontology. Conducting a CGA is feasible in ambulatory geriatric oncology programs (AGOPs) [10,17] including radiation therapy and surgical oncology [18–20]. There are strategies to reduce the time and resources often required to conduct a CGA. The purpose of this article is to illustrate how CGA can be used in different types of AGOPs and is a feasible option despite limited time and personnel. A review of the classic and current literature was conducted using the Ohio State University (OSU) Health Sciences Library (HSL) including PubMed and Cumulative Index to Nursing and Allied Health Literature (CINAHL) to support this article.

1. Defining a Comprehensive Geriatric Assessment

A CGA is a battery of screening tools necessary to uncover actual and potential limitations that can compromise cancer diagnosis and treatment [21]. The Society for International Oncology in

Geriatrics (SIOG) recommends a CGA be administered to older patients who are receiving cancer care [22,23]. Benefits of a CGA are prolonged survival [24], prediction of those who may not benefit from treatment [25], prediction of mortality [26], of cancer treatment tolerance [27], of chemotherapy toxicities [28], of surgical complications [29], and aid in decision-making to help avoid over- and undertreatment of cancer [30]. The battery of screening tools is generally assembled to address common problems associated with aging; however, any number of valid and reliable clinical instruments can be included, depending on the resources. Some cancer centers may be able to conduct large-scale CGA with a robust multidisciplinary team (MDT), and others may limit assessment instruments and MDT members.

The comprehensive character of geriatric assessment allows clinicians to gain perspective beyond the traditional oncology-related history and physical exam [31]. A CGA can detect previously unidentified problems in approximately 70% of patients [32], which can impact cancer treatment [19] and provide the foundation for a treatment plan to address malignant and nonmalignant conditions [33]. CGA is used to develop and refine a cancer management plan specific to the needs of the person diagnosed with cancer [20]. A prime goal of geriatric oncology is helping an older person achieve the best health possible while receiving cancer care to maintain independence [4].

2. Instruments Included in a Comprehensive Geriatric Assessment

Generally, screening tools to detect depression [34], comorbidity [35], cognitive impairment [36], functional status [37,38], risk for falls [39], and nutritional status [40] are commonly included in a CGA. The CGA is multidimensional in that many types of screening instruments can be included to meet the needs of people who are diagnosed with cancer or who are receiving end-of-life care [41], caregivers [42], and providers [43]. SIOG recommends a variety of instruments that can be tailored to any patient population [44].

When choosing instruments to include in a CGA, consider that there are performance-based evaluations and self-report measures. Performance-based evaluations provide a depiction of a person's capability using tools such as the Timed Up and Go Test (TUAGT) [45], balance testing [46], grip strength [47], sit-to-stand test [48], cognitive screening using the Clock Drawing Test [49], and other empirically measured tests. Self-report measures are also commonly included in the CGA, such as the Geriatric Depression Scale (GDS) [34], Activities of Daily Living Scale [37], Instrumental Activities of Daily Living [38], quality-of-life measures [50], and nutritional assessment [40]. Self-report measures tend to be rather easy to use and have validity and reliability metrics for clinical and research use. Including both self-report and performance-based evaluations provides patient perception of functioning at home in conjunction with an objective assessment. Some patients may tend to over-estimate their functional ability, and the empirical observation of task performance may help providers develop realistic management plans.

Supporting the caregiver is also important to the health of the person with cancer [51]. The Modified Caregiver Strain Index [52,53] is a 13-item tool that measures the financial, psychological, personal, physical, and social domains of caregiving which can be incorporated into a CGA. Caregivers of people diagnosed with cancer who have functional impairment [54] and have increased comorbidity [55] report greater strain and burden. CGA can stratify people with cancer into levels of caregiver burden risk so that clinicians can recognize caregivers who may need help [42]. Caregivers of people with advanced cancer often neglect their own health and wellness and report high levels of depression and anxiety [56]. Depression is not rare among caregivers (42%), and clinicians must support and encourage health maintenance and wellness [57]. If caregiver health is not maintained and perceptions of strain and burden exist, the individual with cancer is at risk for re-hospitalization [58] and increased morbidity/mortality [59]. Help for caregivers navigating community resources, Medicare, insurance, and cancer treatment can be very welcomed [60]. Cancer can be overwhelming and expensive, and providing psychosocial support can reduce caregiver stress associated with financial toxicity [61], address depression, and establish coping strategies [62]. No matter the scale of the CGA, caregiver support is important to geriatric oncology.

3. Multidisciplinary Team

A MDT has historically been used in geriatrics to administer the CGA and manage the many interwoven concerns that can affect older people [63,64]. An MDT can be composed of physicians, social workers, pharmacists, nurses, nurse practitioners, dietitians, physical therapists, and other types of healthcare professionals. Not every clinic may have access to a variety of specialists, and it is important to remember that geriatric care and screening can be provided by physicians, nurse practitioners, and nurses. An MDT may simply include a physician and a nurse who are trained in geriatrics. Administering and coordinating a CGA is well within the scope of practice of nursing and can be central to the effectiveness of the MDT [65].

Whatever the size, an MDT functions symbiotically to assess, manage, and monitor many limitations and complications associated with aging and deconditioning [66]. Geriatric oncology has adopted the MDT approach to improve or maintain independence [67] and to provide CGA by which to impact the cancer management plan [20]. Key to an effective MDT are communication, collaboration, and coordination [68]. A social worker, nurse practitioner, and dietitian can evaluate a patient simultaneously and hear the responses from individual assessments, so that questions are not duplicated. This method requires a cohesive teamwork, does save some time, and enhances communication within the MDT. An MDT with a perception of cohesive teamwork provides higher quality of care and less attrition in the nursing staff [69]. Communication with primary care providers and other specialists is critical to geriatric oncology and successful interventions [70]. When primary care providers and oncology providers agree on recommendations, adherence to CGA recommendations is more likely to occur [71].

For providers who lack a MDT, nurse-conducted CGA is a viable option. Nurses and/or advanced practice nurses often function in the role of coordinator, provider, communicator, and organizer. Awareness of the current knowledge in normative aging, geriatric syndromes, wellness, and prevention are components of nursing best practices [72]. Best practices in geriatric/gerontological competencies are provided by the American Association of Colleges of Nursing (AACN) for advanced practice and baccalaureate nurses and largely guide curriculum development for colleges of nursing throughout the United States [73,74]. However, geriatric training is often lacking in nursing schools throughout the country [75], and geriatric education is often received outside of the academic curriculum. The National Hartford Center of Gerontological Nursing Excellence (NHCGNE) aims to enhance gerontological education among nurses in the academic and clinical workforce [76]. The NHCGNE recognizes gerontological nurse educators as *Distinguished Educators in Gerontological Nursing Program* for working with faculty to enhance university and college curricula, educate nursing students at all levels, and work with other providers to better care for the older person [77]. It is important that nurses are educated in gerontology/geriatrics so they are prepared to assess and contribute to the care of the older person who is diagnosed with cancer [78].

4. Management of Problems Detected by Comprehensive Geriatric Assessment

Geriatric syndromes (poor functional status, cognitive impairment, frailty), life expectancy, and comorbidity are realities that oncology providers must consider when caring for older individuals. The mean number of geriatric syndromes is 2.9 in community-dwelling older people [79] and when uncontrolled, may interfere with cancer treatment. Complex problems associated with geriatric syndromes often cannot be addressed in one clinic visit or with a single medication or intervention. For frailer people, determining the cause of a problem may require an MDT-administered CGA and several clinic visits to detect and manage complex problems [80]. Good general health and absence of severe comorbidity allow older people to be considered for surgical [81] and other types of standard treatments [82].

People who have well-managed comorbidities may not have any deterioration in their functional status or life expectancy. In non-metastatic prostate cancer patients receiving treatment, 10-year life expectancy was not impacted by comorbid conditions nor age [83]. However, data show that for every chronic condition, life expectancy decreases 1.8 years [61]. Life expectancy, comorbid conditions, and functional status are sentinel factors in geriatric oncology [84]. Functional status and not chronological age is an important consideration in cancer treatment planning for the older adult [28,85].

Initiating a CGA requires a process to manage the limitations uncovered by the evaluation, and providers should be trained on how to incorporate the MDT recommendations in the decision-making process [86]. The mean number of CGA recommendations to address the uncovered limitations ranges from seven [87] to two [88], depending on the type of patient (frail, vulnerable, or fit) [89]. A CGA performed upon an initial oncology encounter can render three interventions [90]. Patients are most likely to adhere to four or less recommendations unless they present cognitive decline, in which case adherence is lower [87].

Follow-up care is important to determine adherence to recommendations and to reassess the issues that were previously detected [91]. The problems detected in the CGA should be managed or referred and detailed in the medical record [92,93]. How often to administer the CGA depends on the degree of fitness or frailty of the patient. A primary care nurse who is trained in geriatrics can be effective in coordinating the recommendations [94].

5. Comprehensive Geriatric Assessment with Limited Resources

A CGA conducted by an MDT can require an hour or more to administer; however, there are strategies to conduct CGA in a timely and efficient manner. Targeting the person who would most likely benefit from the CGA with a prescreening instrument can help preserve the resources of clinical time and personnel and reduce the respondent burden (Figure 1).

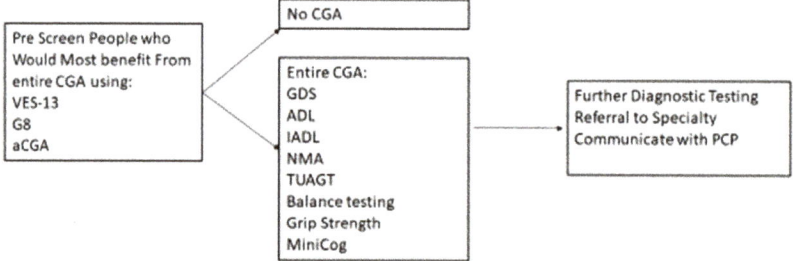

Figure 1. Prescreening using CGA to Determine Further Treatment or Diagnostics.

Prescreens have been developed, such as the abbreviated CGA [95], the G8 [96], and the Vulnerable Elders Survey-13 [97]. SIOG recommends several valid and reliable pre-screen tools [1]. The purpose of pre-screen tools is to target those who most benefit from conducting the entire CGA, rather than to replace a CGA. People who have functional decline and a higher risk of mortality and of cancer treatment complications tend to benefit from the CGA [98,99]. For those people who are independent and with minimal comorbid conditions, a CGA may not be as beneficial [100].

Depending on resources and type of healthcare setting, a CGA can be fashioned to include only several instruments rather than an exhaustive battery of tools requiring hours of clinic encounter time. Creating a smaller version of CGA which can include two or three screening instruments (GDS, Mini-Cog, TUAGT) will allow time to gain experience administering the instrument and managing the limitations. Using only two or three screening instruments has reasonable benefit to people who are diagnosed with cancer and to their families. The detection and management of depression can contribute to better cancer treatment outcomes, particularly with adherence to recommendations [101]. Benefits of screening for cognitive limitations are inconclusive [102]; however, other considerations such as planning, awareness of limitations, preparation for future and other important tasks can be very helpful for patients and families. Screening using the TUAGT can lead to physical therapy consults [88] to enhance lower extremity strength and to provide falls education and proactive planning should a fall occur (determining how to get help, keeping a phone on the bathroom floor near the bathing area). The use of three tools can provide the opportunity to address common problems that can be associated with aging without requiring the time to conduct a more robust CGA (Figure 2).

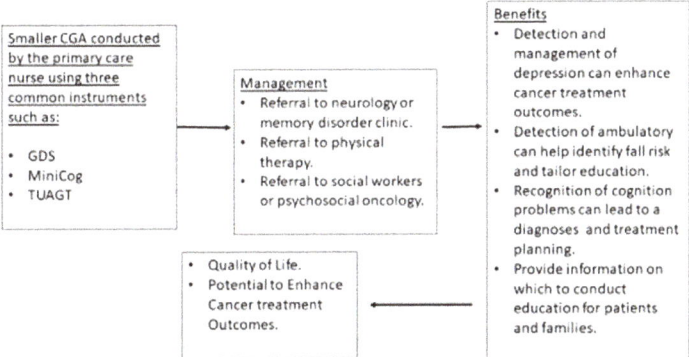

Figure 2. Smaller CGA to Determine Further Treatment or Diagnostics.

The use of pre-screens and a smaller battery of assessment instruments is a viable option when using CGA with limited clinical resources. Understanding the versatility of CGA may motivate more clinicians to employ best practices in geriatric assessment.

Cost and resources are a factor when establishing a geriatric oncology program; however, not all data indicate that CGA is cost-prohibitive when looking at long-term expenses and hospital stay. The SIOG suggests that CGA is cost-effective and reduces hospitalizations [103]. CGA in people who experience a hip fracture reduces hospital costs and hospital length of stay and improves health outcomes [104]. However, for those people admitted to the hospital for nonmalignant conditions, CGA is thought to slightly increase costs [105]. A Swedish study found ambulatory oncology CGA to have increased costs due to the number of interventions and increased survival [25]. Another Swedish study found ambulatory CGA to increase survival in frail people, with fewer hospital days and without higher costs [106]. In the United States, the cost savings or expenses may be different, however, people tend to benefit from CGA [85,107].

6. Models of Geriatric Oncology Programs Using CGA

AGOPs often include regular CGAs and manage a patient throughout cancer care. There are different types of AGOPs, such as those that provide ongoing geriatric oncology management, one-time consult programs, site specific programs, and programs that address patients according to age and not a particular tumor type. Scale also varies among AGOPs, with some using large MDTs and others consisting of an oncologist and a geriatric trained nurse. Regardless of the structure, AGOPs can provide CGA and offer management strategies to enhance the care of the older person diagnosed with cancer.

The CGA can be administered by a nurse or nurse practitioner, and scores on the measures can be shared with the entire MDT, so that more in-depth screening can be conducted by the appropriate specialists. In some situations, the MDT members individually screen new patients to establish a baseline condition prior to cancer treatment. The MDT members can then evaluate the patient as needed throughout cancer treatment. Established patients who have received a baseline CGA can receive regular geriatric assessment screening every 6 months or every year. No data exist on how often to conduct a CGA; however, frail or vulnerable patients may require more frequent screening. The National Comprehensive Cancer Network (NCCN) has established guidelines for using CGA when caring for the older adult [108]. A pre-cancer treatment decision tree addresses how and when to use a prescreening and an entire CGA and how CGA can impact treatment decisions for the patient, family, and provider [108].

Scheduling new and established patients visits for any type of AGOP requires planning for extra time to conduct the CGA. For AGOPs conducting the entire CGA with an MDT in addition to establishing a cancer management plan, a new patient visit may require two hours. For those AGOPs using limited measures in the CGA and a limited MDT, perhaps a 30 min visit is appropriate. One-time CGA consults can be easier to schedule in that all patients tend to receive the same screening instruments and assessment from the MDT. Generally, the consult can be conducted in approximately 1.5 to 2 h per patient. Depending on the physical environment of the clinic, three patients can be scheduled every 2–2.5 hour and be accommodated with rotating members of the team conducting the assessments.

An AGOP one-time CGA consult functions to provide recommendations for cancer treatment, identifies comorbid conditions, and addresses actual and potential risk factors that can affect health and independence. A one-time CGA consult can be helpful to surgical teams to predict complications [109] and post-surgical delirium when administered prior to surgery [110]. A one-time CGA conducted by a geriatrician prior to emergency surgery reduces hospital length of stay by 55 days [111]. Despite the positive contributions of CGA, many surgeons and other providers fail to consult geriatric services [112]. Education on the benefits of CGA in cancer treatment decision-making is critical for all cancer specialties and providers.

Conducting a CGA and incorporating an MDT require infrastructures and administrative support to lay the foundation for a sustainable geriatric oncology. Often, facilities and providers have difficulty launching and maintaining senior adult programs, for many reasons [113]. Patient scheduling to accommodate longer visit times [114], avenues of referral when limitations are found, adapting the medical record to accommodate scores and recommendations are important tasks to address before initiating geriatric assessment [13]. AGOPs require continued evaluation and maintenance to ensure the process of clinic is working well and the MDT is functioning effectively and productively. Regular team meetings can be helpful to discuss assessment process, patients, and research activities. Regular meetings should include administration, office staff who schedule patient visits, as well as people who work with medical records, who can be helpful in establishing highly functioning clinics, especially in big medical centers. MDT meetings prior to geriatric oncology clinic are very useful to review new and established patients.

A prime component of infrastructure is communication with other providers, which is key to the effectiveness of AGOPs. Many providers feel under-utilized in the development of cancer management plans, and communication is often poor between oncologists and primary care providers [94]. Proactive planning to establish avenues of communication to coordinate the CGA recommendations can reduce redundant assessments and increase effectiveness. Follow-up care and adherence to recommendations are likely to be improved with better communication between geriatric MDTs and other providers and typically require organizational modifications for adequate transfer of patient information [115].

Patient referral to an AGOP is also a consideration when establishing a clinic or a process for other oncology providers to refer patients for a one-time CGA consult or ongoing management. Awareness of the AGOP should be created within the organization and the community. Often, community members are not aware of geriatric oncology services, and providing educational symposiums or brief presentations at various sites common to potential patients and families can offer the opportunity to receive a CGA and cancer care.

An AGOP can provide valuable clinical data to enhance the care of the older person diagnosed with cancer. Establishing a research protocol incorporating CGA data can help improve the science of geriatric oncology and establish a foundation for future funding. Select CGA instruments can be useful clinically as well as appropriate for research. Dissemination is critical to geriatric oncology and helps address the importance of CGA in the care of the older person diagnosed with cancer.

7. Conclusions

CGA is a versatile tool that can be integrated into various oncology clinics and specialties to provide the best care for the older person. Integrating a CGA does require administrative support, infrastructure for patient scheduling, MDT involvement, and a great deal of planning. The importance of understanding the needs of older people with cancer and of their caregivers underscores the significance of CGA and inspires a comprehensive view, helpful to make treatment decisions. CGA is the central element of geriatric oncology and the gold standard of practice to meet the needs of older people.

Author Contributions: Individual contributions are as follows: conceptualization, writing original—draft preparation, writing- review and editing draft preparation was performed by J.O., conceptualization writing—review and editing draft preparation was completed by E.K., N.F., C.U. and N.W.

Funding: This research received no external funding.

Acknowledgments: We would like to thank the Stephanie Spielman Comprehensive Breast Cancer for continued support of geriatric oncology and our Senior Adult Oncology Program.

Conflicts of Interest: We have no conflicts of interest to declare.

References

1. Rocque, G.; Azuero, A.; Halilova, K.; Williams, C.; Kenzik, K.; Yagnik, S.K.; Pisu, M. Most Impactful Factors on the Health-Related Quality of Life of a Geriatric Population with Cancer (S769). *J. Pain Symptom Manag.* **2018**, *55*, 694–695. [CrossRef]
2. Hurria, A. Management of Elderly Patients With Cancer. *J. Natl. Compr. Cancer Netw.* **2013**, *11*, 698–701. [CrossRef]
3. Vallet-Regí, M.; Manzano, M.; López, M.C.; Aapro, M.; Barbacid, M.; Guise, T.A.; Balducci, L.; Mena, A.C.; Romero, P.L.O.; Orellana, M.R.; et al. Management of Cancer in the Older Age Person: An Approach to Complex Medical Decisions. *Oncol.* **2017**, *22*, 335–342. [CrossRef] [PubMed]
4. Balducci, L. Treatment of Breast Cancer in Women Older Than 80 Years Is a Complex Task. *J. Oncol. Pr.* **2016**, *12*, 133–134. [CrossRef] [PubMed]
5. Williams, G.R.; Deal, A.M.; Lund, J.L.; Chang, Y.; Muss, H.B.; Pergolotti, M.; Guerard, E.J.; Shachar, S.S.; Wang, Y.; Kenzik, K.; et al. Patient-Reported Comorbidity and Survival in Older Adults with Cancer. *Oncologist* **2018**, *23*, 433–439. [CrossRef]
6. Klepin, H.D.; Pitcher, B.N.; Ballman, K.V.; Kornblith, A.B.; Hurria, A.; Winer, E.P.; Hudis, C.; Cohen, H.J.; Muss, H.B.; Kimmick, G.G.; et al. Comorbidity, Chemotherapy Toxicity, and Outcomes Among Older Women Receiving Adjuvant Chemotherapy for Breast Cancer on a Clinical Trial: CALGB 49907 and CALGB 361004 (Alliance). *J. Oncol. Pr.* **2014**, *10*, e285–e292. [CrossRef] [PubMed]
7. Kim, K.H.; Lee, J.J.; Kim, J.; Zhou, J.-M.; Gomes, F.; Sehovic, M.; Extermann, M. Association of multidimensional comorbidities with survival, toxicity, and unplanned hospitalizations in older adults with metastatic colorectal cancer treated with chemotherapy. *J. Geriatr. Oncol.* **2019**. [CrossRef]
8. Mariano, C.; Williams, G.; Deal, A.; Alston, S.; Bryant, A.L.; Jolly, T.; Muss, H.B. Geriatric Assessment of Older Adults With Cancer During Unplanned Hospitalizations: An Opportunity in Disguise. *Oncol.* **2015**, *20*, 767–772. [CrossRef]
9. Tjong, M.C.; Menjak, I.; Trudeau, M.; Mehta, R.; Wright, F.; Leahey, A.; Ellis, J.; Gallagher, D.; Gibson, L.; Bristow, B.; et al. Perceptions and Expectations of Older Women in the Establishment of the Senior Women's Breast Cancer Clinic (SWBCC): A Needs Assessment Study. *J. Cancer Educ.* **2017**, *32*, 850–857. [CrossRef]
10. Magnuson, A.; Dale, W.; Mohile, S. Models of Care in Geriatric Oncology. *Curr. Geriatr. Rep.* **2014**, *3*, 182–189. [CrossRef]
11. O'Donovan, A.; Leech, M.; Mohile, S. Expert consensus panel guidelines on geriatric assessment in oncology. *Eur. J. Cancer Care* **2015**, *24*, 574–589. [CrossRef] [PubMed]

12. Burhenn, P.S.; Perrin, S.; McCarthy, A.L.; Information, P.E.K.F.C. Models of Care in Geriatric Oncology Nursing. *Semin. Oncol. Nurs.* **2016**, *32*, 24–32. [CrossRef] [PubMed]
13. Overcash, J. Integrating Geriatrics Into Oncology Ambulatory Care Clinics. *Clin. J. Oncol. Nurs.* **2015**, *19*, E80–E86. [CrossRef] [PubMed]
14. Goede, V.; Stauder, R. Multidisciplinary care in the hematology clinic: Implementation of geriatric oncology. *J. Geriatr. Oncol.* **2018**, *10*, 497–503. [CrossRef] [PubMed]
15. Chapman, A.E.; Swartz, K.; Schoppe, J.; Arenson, C. Development of a comprehensive multidisciplinary geriatric oncology center, the Thomas Jefferson University Experience. *J. Geriatr. Oncol.* **2014**, *5*, 164–170. [CrossRef]
16. Le Saux, O.; Falandry, C.; Gan, H.K.; You, B.; Freyer, G.; Péron, J. Changes in the Use of Comprehensive Geriatric Assessment in Clinical Trials for Older Patients with Cancer over Time. *Oncol.* **2019**. [CrossRef] [PubMed]
17. Puts, M.T.E.; Hardt, J.; Monette, J.; Girre, V.; Springall, E.; Alibhai, S.M.H. Use of Geriatric Assessment for Older Adults in the Oncology Setting: A Systematic Review. *J. Natl. Cancer Inst.* **2012**, *104*, 1134–1164. [CrossRef] [PubMed]
18. Szumacher, E.; Sattar, S.; Neve, M.; Do, K.; Ayala, A.; Gray, M.; Lee, J.; Alibhai, S.; Puts, M. Use of Comprehensive Geriatric Assessment and Geriatric Screening for Older Adults in the Radiation Oncology Setting: A Systematic Review. *Clin. Oncol.* **2018**, *30*, 578–588. [CrossRef]
19. Alibhai, S.M.; Jin, R.; Loucks, A.; Yokom, D.W.; Watt, S.; Puts, M.; Timilshina, N.; Berger, A. Beyond the black box of geriatric assessment: Understanding enhancements to care by the geriatric oncology clinic. *J. Geriatr. Oncol.* **2018**, *9*, 679–682. [CrossRef]
20. Festen, S.; Kok, M.; Hopstaken, J.S.; van der Wal-Huisman, H.; van der Leest, A.; Reyners, A.K.L.; de Bock, G.H.; de Graeff, P.; van Leeuwen, B.L. How to incorporate geriatric assessment in clinical decision-making for older patients with cancer. An implementation study. *J. Geriatr. Oncol.* **2019**. [CrossRef]
21. Solomon, D. National Institutes of Health Consensus Development Conference Statement: Geriatric Assessment Methods for Clinical Decision-Making. *Am. Geriatr. Soc.* **1988**, *36*, 342–437.
22. Wildiers, H.; Heeren, P.; Puts, M.; Topinkova, E.; Janssen-Heijnen, M.L.; Extermann, M.; Falandry, C.; Artz, A.; Brain, E.; Colloca, G.; et al. International Society of Geriatric Oncology Consensus on Geriatric Assessment in Older Patients With Cancer. *J. Clin. Oncol.* **2014**, *32*, 2595–2603. [CrossRef] [PubMed]
23. Mohile, S.G.; Velarde, C.; Hurria, A.; Magnuson, A.; Lowenstein, L.; Pandya, C.; O'Donovan, A.; Gorawara-Bhat, R.; Dale, W. Geriatric Assessment-Guided Care Processes for Older Adults: A Delphi Consensus of Geriatric Oncology Experts. *J. Natl. Compr. Cancer Netw.* **2015**, *13*, 1120–1130. [CrossRef]
24. Kenis, C.; Baitar, A.; DeCoster, L.; De Grève, J.; Lobelle, J.-P.; Flamaing, J.; Milisen, K.; Wildiers, H. The added value of geriatric screening and assessment for predicting overall survival in older patients with cancer. *Cancer* **2018**, *124*, 3753–3763. [CrossRef] [PubMed]
25. Lundqvist, M.; Alwin, J.; Henriksson, M.; Husberg, M.; Carlsson, P.; Ekdahl, A.W. Cost-effectiveness of comprehensive geriatric assessment at an ambulatory geriatric unit based on the AGe-FIT trial. *BMC Geriatr.* **2018**, *18*, 32. [CrossRef] [PubMed]
26. Hamaker, M.E.; Vos, A.G.; Smorenburg, C.H.; De Rooij, S.E.; Van Munster, B.C. The Value of Geriatric Assessments in Predicting Treatment Tolerance and All-Cause Mortality in Older Patients With Cancer. *Oncol.* **2012**, *17*, 1439–1449. [CrossRef] [PubMed]
27. Freyer, G.; Geay, J.-F.; Touzet, S.; Provencal, J.; Weber, B.; Jacquin, J.-P.; Ganem, G.; Mathieu, N.T.; Gisserot, O.; Pujade-Lauraine, E. Comprehensive geriatric assessment predicts tolerance to chemotherapy and survival in elderly patients with advanced ovarian carcinoma: A GINECO study. *Ann. Oncol.* **2005**, *16*, 1795–1800. [CrossRef] [PubMed]
28. Soto-Perez-De-Celis, E.; Li, D.; Yuan, Y.; Lau, Y.M.; Hurria, A. Functional versus chronological age: Geriatric assessments to guide decision making in older patients with cancer. *Lancet Oncol.* **2018**, *19*, e305–e316. [CrossRef]
29. Kristjansson, S.R.; Nesbakken, A.; Jordhøy, M.S.; Skovlund, E.; Audisio, R.A.; Johannessen, H.-O.; Bakka, A.; Wyller, T.B. Comprehensive geriatric assessment can predict complications in elderly patients after elective surgery for colorectal cancer: A prospective observational cohort study. *Crit. Rev. Oncol.* **2010**, *76*, 208–217. [CrossRef]

30. Schiphorst, A.H.; Ten Bokkel Huinink, D.; Breumelhof, R.; Burgmans, J.P.; Pronk, A.; Hamaker, M.E. Geriatric consultation can aid in complex treatment decisions for elderly cancer patients. *Eur. J. Cancer Care (Engl.)* **2016**, *25*, 365–370. [CrossRef]
31. Caillet, P.; Laurent, M.; Bastuji-Garin, S.; Liuu, E.; Culine, S.; Lagrange, J.-L.; Canoui-Poitrine, F.; Paillaud, E. Optimal management of elderly cancer patients: Usefulness of the Comprehensive Geriatric Assessment. *Clin. Interv. Aging* **2014**, *9*, 1645–1660. [PubMed]
32. Horgan, A.M.; Leighl, N.B.; Coate, L.; Liu, G.; Palepu, P.; Knox, J.J.; Perera, N.; Emami, M.; Alibhai, S.M. Impact and feasibility of a comprehensive geriatric assessment in the oncology setting: A pilot study. *Am. J. Clin. Oncol.* **2012**, *35*, 322–328. [CrossRef] [PubMed]
33. Hamaker, M.E.; Molder, M.T.; Thielen, N.; Van Munster, B.C.; Schiphorst, A.H.; Van Huis, L.H. The effect of a geriatric evaluation on treatment decisions and outcome for older cancer patients – A systematic review. *J. Geriatr. Oncol.* **2018**, *9*, 430–440. [CrossRef] [PubMed]
34. Yesavage, J.A.; Brink, T.; Rose, T.L.; Lum, O.; Huang, V.; Adey, M.; Leirer, V.O. Development and validation of a geriatric depression screening scale: A preliminary report. *J. Psychiatr. Res.* **1982**, *17*, 37–49. [CrossRef]
35. Charlson, M.E.; Pompei, P.; Ales, K.L.; MacKenzie, C. A new method of classifying prognostic comorbidity in longitudinal studies: Development and validation. *J. Chronic Dis.* **1987**, *40*, 373–383. [CrossRef]
36. Borson, S.; Scanlan, J.; Brush, M.; Vitaliano, P.; Dokmak, A. The Mini-Cog: A cognitive "vital signs" measure for dementia screening in multi-lingual elderly. *Int. J. Geriatr. Psychiatry* **2000**, *15*, 1021–1027. [CrossRef]
37. Katz, S.; Grotz, R.C.; Downs, T.D.; Cash, H.R. Progress in Development of the Index of ADL. *Gerontol.* **1970**, *10*, 20–30. [CrossRef] [PubMed]
38. Lawton, M.P.; Brody, E.M. Assessment of Older People: Self-Maintaining and Instrumental Activities of Daily Living. *Gerontol.* **1969**, *9*, 179–186. [CrossRef]
39. Kellogg International Work Group. A report of the Kellogg International Work Group on the Prevention of Falls by the Elderly. *Dan. Med. Bull.* **1987**, *34* (Suppl. 4), 1–24.
40. Vellas, B.; Guigoz, Y.; Garry, P.J.; Nourhashemi, F.; Bennahum, D.; Lauque, S.; Albarède, J.-L. The mini nutritional assessment (MNA) and its use in grading the nutritional state of elderly patients. *Nutr.* **1999**, *15*, 116–122. [CrossRef]
41. Baronner, A.; MacKenzie, A. Using Geriatric Assessment Strategies to Lead End-of-Life Care Discussions. *Curr. Oncol. Rep.* **2017**, *19*. [CrossRef] [PubMed]
42. Rajasekaran, T.; Tan, T.; Ong, W.S.; Koo, K.N.; Chan, L.; Poon, D.; Chowdhury, A.R.; Krishna, L.; Kanesvaran, R.; Information, P.E.K.F.C. Comprehensive Geriatric Assessment (CGA) based risk factors for increased caregiver burden among elderly Asian patients with cancer. *J. Geriatr. Oncol.* **2016**, *7*, 211–218. [CrossRef] [PubMed]
43. Hamaker, M.; Seynaeve, C.; Wymenga, A.; Van Tinteren, H.; Nortier, J.; Maartense, E.; De Graaf, H.; De Jongh, F.; Braun, J.; Los, M.; et al. Baseline comprehensive geriatric assessment is associated with toxicity and survival in elderly metastatic breast cancer patients receiving single-agent chemotherapy: Results from the OMEGA study of the Dutch Breast Cancer Trialists' Group. *Breast* **2014**, *23*, 81–87. [CrossRef] [PubMed]
44. International Society of Oncology Geraitrics. Comprehensive Geraitric Assessment of the Older Person with Cancer. 2015. Available online: http://www.siog.org/content/comprehensive-geriatric-assessment-cga-older-patient-cancer (accessed on 11 June 2019).
45. Podsiadlo, D.; Richardson, S. The Timed "Up & Go": A Test of Basic Functional Mobility for Frail Elderly Persons. *J. Am. Geriatr. Soc.* **1991**, *39*, 142–148. [PubMed]
46. Berg, K.O.; Wood-Dauphinee, S.L.; Williams, J.I.; Maki, B. Measuring balance in the elderly: Validation of an instrument. *Can. J. Public Heal.* **1992**, *83*, S7–S11.
47. Mathiowetz, V.; Weber, K.; Volland, G.; Kashman, N. Reliability and validity of grip and pinch strength evaluations. *J. Hand Surg.* **1984**, *9*, 222–226. [CrossRef]
48. Jones, C.J.; Rikli, R.E.; Beam, W.C. A 30-s Chair-Stand Test as a Measure of Lower Body Strength in Community-Residing Older Adults. *Res. Q. Exerc. Sport* **1999**, *70*, 113–119. [CrossRef]
49. Borson, S.; Brush, M.; Gil, E.; Scanlan, J.; Vitaliano, P.; Chen, J.; Cashman, J.; Maria, M.M.S.; Barnhart, R.; Roques, J. The Clock Drawing Test: Utility for Dementia Detection in Multiethnic Elders. *Journals Gerontol. Ser. A: Boil. Sci. Med Sci.* **1999**, *54*, M534–M540. [CrossRef]
50. Cella, D.F.; Tulsky, D.S.; Gray, G.; Sarafian, B.; Linn, E.; Bonomi, A.; Silberman, M.; Yellen, S.B.; Winicour, P.; Brannon, J. The Functional Assessment of Cancer Therapy scale: Development and validation of the general measure. *J. Clin. Oncol.* **1993**, *11*, 570–579. [CrossRef]

51. Sakurai, R.; Kawai, H.; Suzuki, H.; Kim, H.; Watanabe, Y.; Hirano, H.; Ihara, K.; Obuchi, S.; Fujiwara, Y. Poor Social Network, Not Living Alone, Is Associated With Incidence of Adverse Health Outcomes in Older Adults. *J. Am. Med Dir. Assoc.* **2019**. [CrossRef]
52. Thornton, M.; Travis, S.S. Analysis of the Reliability of the Modified Caregiver Strain Index. *Journals Gerontol. Ser. B* **2003**, *58*, S127–S132. [CrossRef] [PubMed]
53. Robinson, B.C. Validation of a Caregiver Strain Index. *J. Gerontol.* **1983**, *38*, 344–348. [CrossRef] [PubMed]
54. Bień-Barkowska, K.; Doroszkiewicz, H.; Bień, B. Silent strain of caregiving: Exploring the best predictors of distress in family carers of geriatric patients. *Clin. Interv. Aging* **2017**, *12*, 263–274. [CrossRef] [PubMed]
55. Dauphinot, V.; Ravier, A.; Novais, T.; Delphin-Combe, F.; Moutet, C.; Xie, J.; Mouchoux, C.; Krolak-Salmon, P.; Information, P.E.K.F.C. Relationship Between Comorbidities in Patients With Cognitive Complaint and Caregiver Burden: A Cross-Sectional Study. *J. Am. Med Dir. Assoc.* **2016**, *17*, 232–237. [CrossRef]
56. Dionne-Odom, J.N.; Demark-Wahnefried, W.; Taylor, R.A.; Rocque, G.B.; Azuero, A.; Acemgil, A.; Martin, M.Y.; Astin, M.; Ejem, D.; Kvale, E.; et al. The Self-Care Practices of Family Caregivers of Persons with Poor Prognosis Cancer: Differences by Varying Levels of Caregiver Well-being and Preparedness. *Support. Care Cancer* **2017**, *25*, 2437–2444. [CrossRef] [PubMed]
57. Geng, H.M.; Chuang, D.M.; Yang, F.; Yang, Y.; Liu, W.M.; Liu, L.H.; Tian, H.M. Prevalence and determinants of depression in caregivers of cancer patients: A systematic review and meta-analysis. *Medicine (Baltimore)* **2018**, *97*, e11863. [CrossRef]
58. Bonin-Guillaume, S.; Durand, A.-C.; Yahi, F.; Curiel-Berruyer, M.; Lacroix, O.; Cretel, E.; Alazia, M.; Sambuc, R.; Gentile, S. Predictive factors for early unplanned rehospitalization of older adults after an ED visit: Role of the caregiver burden. *Aging Clin. Exp. Res.* **2015**, *27*, 883–891. [CrossRef] [PubMed]
59. Aggarwal, B.; Liao, M.; Christian, A.; Mosca, L. Influence of caregiving on lifestyle and psychosocial risk factors among family members of patients hospitalized with cardiovascular disease. *J. Gen. Intern. Med.* **2009**, *24*, 93–98. [CrossRef]
60. Lawn, S.; Westwood, T.; Jordans, S.; O'Connor, J. Support workers as agents for health behavior change: An Australian study of the perceptions of clients with complex needs, support workers, and care coordinators. *Gerontol. Geriatr. Educ.* **2017**, *38*, 496–516. [CrossRef]
61. DuGoff, E.H.; Canudas-Romo, V.; Buttorff, C.; Leff, B.; Anderson, G.F. Multiple chronic conditions and life expectancy: A life table analysis. *Med. Care* **2014**, *52*, 688–694. [CrossRef]
62. Nelson, C.J.; Saracino, R.M.; Roth, A.J.; Harvey, E.; Martin, A.; Moore, M.; Marcone, D.; Poppito, S.R.; Holland, J. Cancer and Aging: Reflections for Elders (CARE): A pilot randomized controlled trial of a psychotherapy intervention for older adults with cancer. *Psychooncology* **2019**, *28*, 39–47. [CrossRef] [PubMed]
63. Rubenstein, L.Z.; Josephson, K.R.; Wieland, G.D.; English, P.A.; Sayre, J.A.; Kane, R.L. Effectiveness of a Geriatric Evaluation Unit. *New Engl. J. Med.* **1984**, *311*, 1664–1670. [CrossRef] [PubMed]
64. Warren, M.W. Care of Chronic Sick. *Br. Med. J.* **1943**, *2*, 822–823. [CrossRef] [PubMed]
65. Trotta, R.L.; Rao, A.D.; Hermann, R.M.; Boltz, M.P. Development of a Comprehensive Geriatric Assessment Led by Geriatric Nurse Consultants: A Feasibility Study. *J. Gerontol. Nurs.* **2018**, *44*, 25–34. [CrossRef] [PubMed]
66. Flood, K.L.; Booth, K.; Vickers, J.; Simmons, E.; James, D.H.; Biswal, S.; Deaver, J.; White, M.L.; Bowman, E.H. Acute Care for Elders (ACE) Team Model of Care: A Clinical Overview. *Geriatr.* **2018**, *3*, 50. [CrossRef] [PubMed]
67. Balducci, L.; Yates, J. General guidelines for the management of older patients with cancer. *Oncol. (Williston Park. N.Y.)* **2000**, *14*, 221–227.
68. Karnakis, T.; Gattas-Vernaglia, I.F.; Saraiva, M.D.; Gil-Junior, L.A.; Kanaji, A.L.; Jacob-Filho, W. The geriatrician's perspective on practical aspects of the multidisciplinary care of older adults with cancer. *J. Geriatr. Oncol.* **2016**, *7*, 341–345. [CrossRef] [PubMed]
69. Piers, R.D.; Versluys, K.; Devoghel, J.; Vyt, A.; Noortgate, N.V.D. Interprofessional teamwork, quality of care and turnover intention in geriatric care: A cross-sectional study in 55 acute geriatric units. *Int. J. Nurs. Stud.* **2019**, *91*, 94–100. [CrossRef]
70. Nazir, A.; Unroe, K.; Tegeler, M.; Khan, B.; Azar, J.; Boustani, M. Systematic Review of Interdisciplinary Interventions in Nursing Homes. *J. Am. Med Dir. Assoc.* **2013**, *14*, 471–478. [CrossRef]

71. Maly, R.C.; Leake, B.; Frank, J.C.; DiMatteo, M.R.; Reuben, D.B. Implementation of consultative geriatric recommendations: The role of patient-primary care physician concordance. *J. Am. Geriatr. Soc.* **2002**, *50*, 1372–1380. [CrossRef]
72. McConnell, E.S.; Lekan, D.; Bunn, M.; Egerton, E.; Corazzini, K.N.; Hendrix, C.D.; E Bailey, D. Teaching evidence-based nursing practice in geriatric care settings: The geriatric nursing innovations through education institute. *J. Gerontol. Nurs.* **2009**, *35*, 26–33. [PubMed]
73. American Assocaition of Colleges of Nursing. Adult Gerontology Acute Care and Primary Care Competencies. 2016. Available online: http://www.aacnnursing.org/Portals/42/AcademicNursing/pdf/Adult-Gero-NP-Comp-2016.pdf (accessed on 20 June 2019).
74. American Nurses Credentialing Center. Gerontological Nursing Certification. 2018. Available online: https://www.nursingworld.org/our-certifications/gerontological-nurse/ (accessed on 20 June 2019).
75. Gilje, F.; Lacey, L.; Moore, C. Gerontology and Geriatric Issues and Trends in U.S. Nursing Programs: A National Survey. *J. Prof. Nurs.* **2007**, *23*, 21–29. [CrossRef] [PubMed]
76. Bednash, G.; Mezey, M.; Tagliareni, E. The Hartford Geriatric Nursing Initiative experience in geriatric nursing education: Looking back, looking forward. *Nurs. Outlook* **2011**, *59*, 228–235. [CrossRef] [PubMed]
77. National Hartford Center of Nursing Excellence. Distinguished Educator in Gerontological Nursing. 2018. Available online: https://www.nhcgne.org/leadership-development/distinguished-educator-in-gerontological-nursing-program (accessed on 18 May 2019).
78. Burhenn, P.S.; McCarthy, A.L.; Begue, A.; Nightingale, G.; Cheng, K.; Kenis, C. Geriatric assessment in daily oncology practice for nurses and allied health care professionals: Opinion paper of the Nursing and Allied Health Interest Group of the International Society of Geriatric Oncology (SIOG). *J. Geriatr. Oncol.* **2016**, *7*, 315–324. [CrossRef] [PubMed]
79. Tkacheva, O.N.; Runikhina, N.K.; Ostapenko, V.S.; Sharashkina, N.V.; A Mkhitaryan, E.; Onuchina, J.S.; Lysenkov, S.N.; Yakhno, N.N.; Press, Y. Prevalence of geriatric syndromes among people aged 65 years and older at four community clinics in Moscow. *Clin. Interv. Aging* **2018**, *13*, 251–259. [CrossRef] [PubMed]
80. Overcash, J.; Cope, D.G.; Van Cleave, J.H. Frailty in Older Adults: Assessment, Support, and Treatment Implications in Patients With Cancer. *Clin. J. Oncol. Nurs.* **2018**, *22*, 8–18.
81. Banysch, M.; Akkaya, T.; Gurenko, P.; Papadakis, M.; Heuer, T.; Kasim, E.; Tavarajah, S.S.; Kaiser, G.M. Surgery for colorectal cancer in elderly patients: Is there such a thing as being too old? *G Chir* **2018**, *39*, 355–362.
82. Vitale, S.G.; Capriglione, S.; Zito, G.; Lopez, S.; Gulino, F.A.; Di Guardo, F.; Vitagliano, A.; Noventa, M.; La Rosa, V.L.; Sapia, F.; et al. Management of endometrial, ovarian and cervical cancer in the elderly: Current approach to a challenging condition. *Arch. Gynecol. Obstet.* **2019**, *299*, 299–315. [CrossRef]
83. Boehm, K.; Dell'Oglio, P.; Tian, Z.; Capitanio, U.; Chun, F.K.H.; Tilki, D.; Haferkamp, A.; Saad, F.; Montorsi, F.; Graefen, M.; et al. Comorbidity and age cannot explain variation in life expectancy associated with treatment of non-metastatic prostate cancer. *World J. Urol.* **2017**, *35*, 1031–1036. [CrossRef]
84. Shachar, S.S.; Hurria, A.; Muss, H.B. Breast Cancer in Women Older Than 80 Years. *J. Oncol. Pr.* **2016**, *12*, 123–132. [CrossRef]
85. Droz, J.-P.; Boyle, H.; Albrand, G.; Mottet, N.; Puts, M. Role of Geriatric Oncologists in Optimizing Care of Urological Oncology Patients. *Eur. Urol. Focus* **2017**, *3*, 385–394. [CrossRef] [PubMed]
86. Sarrió, R.G.; On behalf of the Spanish Working Group on Geriatric Oncology of the Spanish Society of Medical Oncology (SEOM); Rebollo, M.A.; Garrido, M.J.M.; Guillen-Ponce, C.; Blanco, R.; Flores, E.G.; Saldaña, J. General recommendations paper on the management of older patients with cancer: The SEOM geriatric oncology task force's position statement. *Clin. Transl. Oncol.* **2018**, *20*, 1246–1251.
87. Morin, T.; Lanièce, I.; Desbois, A.; Amiard, S.; Gavazzi, G.; Couturier, P. Evaluation of adherence to recommendations within 3 months after comprehensive geriatric assessment by an inpatient geriatric consultation team. *Geriatr Psychol Neuropsychiatr Vieil* **2012**, *10*, 285–293. [PubMed]
88. Overcash, J. Comprehensive Geriatric Assessment: Interprofessional Team Recommendations for Older Adult Women With Breast Cancer. *Clin. J. Oncol. Nurs.* **2018**, *22*, 304–315. [CrossRef] [PubMed]
89. Balducci, L. Frailty: A Common Pathway in Aging and Cancer. *Primate Reproductive Aging* **2013**, *38*, 61–72.
90. Boulahssass, R.; Gonfrier, S.; Champigny, N.; Lassalle, S.; François, E.; Hofman, P.; Guerin, O. The Desire to Better Understand Older Adults with Solid Tumors to Improve Management: Assessment and Guided Interventions—The French PACA EST Cohort Experience. *Cancers* **2019**, *11*, 192. [CrossRef] [PubMed]

91. Extermann, M.; Aapro, M.; Bernabei, R.; Cohen, H.J.; Droz, J.P.; Lichtman, S.; Topinkova, E. Use of comprehensive geriatric assessment in older cancer patients: Recommendations from the task force on CGA of the International Society of Geriatric Oncology (SIOG). *Crit. Rev. Oncol. Hematol.* **2005**, *55*, 241–252. [CrossRef]
92. Mohile, S.G.; Dale, W.; Somerfield, M.R.; Schonberg, M.A.; Boyd, C.M.; Burhenn, P.S.; Canin, B.; Cohen, H.J.; Holmes, H.M.; Hopkins, J.O.; et al. Practical Assessment and Management of Vulnerabilities in Older Patients Receiving Chemotherapy: ASCO Guideline for Geriatric Oncology. *J. Clin. Oncol.* **2018**, *36*, 2326–2347. [CrossRef]
93. Verweij, N.M.; Souwer, E.T.D.; Schiphorst, A.H.W.; Maas, H.A.; Portielje, J.E.A.; Pronk, A.; Bos, F.V.D.; Hamaker, M.E. The effect of a geriatric evaluation on treatment decisions for older patients with colorectal cancer. *Int. J. Color. Dis.* **2017**, *32*, 1625–1629. [CrossRef]
94. Puts, M.T.; Strohschein, F.J.; Del Giudice, M.E.; Jin, R.; Loucks, A.; Ayala, A.P.; Alibhai, S.H. Role of the geriatrician, primary care practitioner, nurses, and collaboration with oncologists during cancer treatment delivery for older adults: A narrative review of the literature. *J. Geriatr. Oncol.* **2018**, *9*, 398–404. [CrossRef]
95. Overcash, J.A.; Beckstead, J.; Extermann, M.; Cobb, S. The abbreviated comprehensive geriatric assessment (aCGA): A retrospective analysis. *Crit. Rev. Oncol.* **2005**, *54*, 129–136. [CrossRef]
96. Soubeyran, P.-L.; Bellera, C.; Goyard, J.; Heitz, D.; Curé, H.; Rousselot, H.; Albrand, G.; Servent, V.; Jean, O.S.; Van Praagh, I.; et al. Screening for Vulnerability in Older Cancer Patients: The ONCODAGE Prospective Multicenter Cohort Study. *PLOS ONE* **2014**, *9*, 115060. [CrossRef] [PubMed]
97. Mohile, S.G.; Bylow, K.; Dale, W.; Dignam, J.; Martin, K.; Petrylak, D.P.; Stadler, W.M.; Rodin, M. A pilot study of the vulnerable elders survey-13 compared with the comprehensive geriatric assessment for identifying disability in older patients with prostate cancer who receive androgen ablation. *Cancer* **2007**, *109*, 802–810. [CrossRef] [PubMed]
98. Torres, C.H.; Hsu, T. Comprehensive Geriatric Assessment in the Older Adult with Cancer: A Review. *Eur. Urol. Focus* **2017**, *3*, 330–339. [CrossRef] [PubMed]
99. Locher, C.; Pourel, N.; Le Caer, H.; Bérard, H.; Auliac, J.-B.; Monnet, I.; Descourt, R.; Vergnenègre, A.; Lafay, I.M.; Greillier, L.; et al. Impact of a comprehensive geriatric assessment to manage elderly patients with locally advanced non-small-cell lung cancers: An open phase II study using concurrent cisplatin–oral vinorelbine and radiotherapy (GFPC 08-06). *Lung Cancer* **2018**, *121*, 25–29. [CrossRef]
100. Palmer, K.; Onder, G. Comprehensive geriatric assessment: Benefits and limitations. *Eur. J. Intern. Med.* **2018**, *54*, e8–e9. [CrossRef] [PubMed]
101. Decker, V.; Sikorskii, A.; Given, C.W.; Given, B.A.; Vachon, E.; Krauss, J.C. Effects of depressive symptomatology on cancer-related symptoms during oral oncolytic treatment. *Psychooncology* **2019**, *28*, 99–106. [CrossRef]
102. Moyer, V.A.; Force, U.P.S.T. Screening for cognitive impairment in older adults: U.S. Preventive Services Task Force recommendation statement. *Ann. Intern. Med.* **2014**, *160*, 791–797. [CrossRef]
103. Extermann, M. Geriatric Assessment with Focus on Instrument Selectivity for Outcomes. *Cancer J.* **2005**, *11*, 474–480. [CrossRef]
104. Eamer, G.; Saravana-Bawan, B.; Van Der Westhuizen, B.; Chambers, T.; Ohinmaa, A.; Khadaroo, R.G. Economic evaluations of comprehensive geriatric assessment in surgical patients: A systematic review. *J. Surg. Res.* **2017**, *218*, 9–17. [CrossRef]
105. Gardner, M.; Tsiachristas, A.; Langhorne, P.; Burke, O.; Harwood, R.H.; Conroy, S.P.; Kircher, T.; Somme, D.; Saltvedt, I.; Wald, H.; et al. Comprehensive geriatric assessment for older adults admitted to hospital. *Cochrane Database Syst. Rev.* **2017**, *2017*, CD006211.
106. Ekdahl, A.W.; Alwin, J.; Eckerblad, J.; Husberg, M.; Jaarsma, T.; Mazya, A.L.; Milberg, A.; Krevers, B.; Unosson, M.; Wiklund, R.; et al. Long-Term Evaluation of the Ambulatory Geriatric Assessment: A Frailty Intervention Trial (AGe-FIT): Clinical Outcomes and Total Costs After 36 Months. *J. Am. Med. Dir. Assoc.* **2016**, *17*, 263–268. [CrossRef] [PubMed]
107. Bhatt, V.R. Personalizing therapy for older adults with acute myeloid leukemia: Role of geriatric assessment and genetic profiling. *Cancer Treat. Rev.* **2019**, *75*, 52–61. [CrossRef]
108. NCCN. *Clinical Practice Guidelines in Oncology: Older Adult Oncology*; NCCN: Plymouth Meeting, PA, USA, 2019.

109. Xue, D.-D.; Cheng, Y.; Wu, M.; Zhang, Y. Comprehensive geriatric assessment prediction of postoperative complications in gastrointestinal cancer patients: A meta-analysis. *Clin. Interv. Aging* **2018**, *13*, 723–736. [CrossRef] [PubMed]
110. Maekawa, Y.; Sugimoto, K.; Yamasaki, M.; Takeya, Y.; Yamamoto, K.; Ohishi, M.; Ogihara, T.; Shintani, A.; Doki, Y.; Mori, M.; et al. Comprehensive Geriatric Assessment is a useful predictive tool for postoperative delirium after gastrointestinal surgery in old-old adults. *Geriatr. Gerontol. Int.* **2016**, *16*, 1036–1042. [CrossRef] [PubMed]
111. Mason, M.C.; Crees, A.L.; Dean, M.R.; Bashir, N. Establishing a proactive geriatrician led comprehensive geriatric assessment in older emergency surgery patients: Outcomes of a pilot study. *Int. J. Clin. Pr.* **2018**, *72*, e13096. [CrossRef] [PubMed]
112. Ghignone, F.; Van Leeuwen, B.; Montroni, I.; Huisman, M.; Somasundar, P.; Cheung, K.; Audisio, R.; Ugolini, G. The assessment and management of older cancer patients: A SIOG surgical task force survey on surgeons' attitudes. *Eur. J. Surg. Oncol. (EJSO)* **2016**, *42*, 297–302. [CrossRef]
113. To, T.H.M.; Soo, W.K.; Lane, H.; Khattak, A.; Steer, C.; Devitt, B.; Dhillon, H.M.; Booms, A.; Phillips, J. Utilization of geriatric assessment in oncology—A survey of Australian medical oncologists. *J. Geriatr. Oncol.* **2019**, *10*, 216–221. [CrossRef]
114. Koneru, R.; Freedman, O.; Lemonde, M.; Froese, J. Evaluation of a comprehensive geriatric assessment tool in geriatric cancer patients undergoing adjuvant chemotherapy: A pilot study. *Support. Care Cancer* **2019**, *27*, 1871–1877. [CrossRef]
115. Kagan, E.; Freud, T.; Punchik, B.; Barzak, A.; Peleg, R.; Press, Y.A. Comparative Study of Models of Geriatric Assessment and the Implementation of Recommendations by Primary Care Physicians. *Rejuvenation Res.* **2017**, *20*, 278–285. [CrossRef]

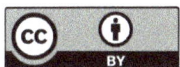

© 2019 by the authors. Licensee MDPI, Basel, Switzerland. This article is an open access article distributed under the terms and conditions of the Creative Commons Attribution (CC BY) license (http://creativecommons.org/licenses/by/4.0/).

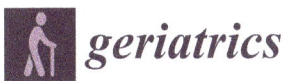

Article

Evaluation of a Combined HIV and Geriatrics Clinic for Older People Living with HIV: The Silver Clinic in Brighton, UK

Tom Levett [1,2], Katie Alford [3], Jonathan Roberts [1], Zoe Adler [1], Juliet Wright [1,4] and Jaime H. Vera [1,3,*]

1. Division of Medicine, Brighton and Sussex University Hospitals NHS Trust, UK; t.levett@nhs.net (T.L.); jonathan.roberts10@nhs.net (J.R.); zoe.adler@nhs.net (Z.A.); juliet.wright6@nhs.net (J.W.)
2. Department of Clinical and Experimental Medicine, Brighton and Sussex Medical School, Falmer, Brighton BN1 9PX, UK
3. Department of Global Health and Infection, Brighton and Sussex Medical School, Falmer, Brighton BN1 9PX, UK; K.Alford2@bsms.ac.uk
4. Department of Medical Education, Brighton and Sussex Medical School, Falmer, Brighton BN1 9PX, UK
* Correspondence: j.vera@bsms.ac.uk

Received: 11 August 2020; Accepted: 13 October 2020; Published: 19 October 2020

Abstract: As life expectancy in people living with HIV (PLWH) has increased, the focus of management has shifted to preventing and treating chronic illnesses, but few services exist for the assessment and management of these individuals. Here, we provide an initial description of a geriatric service for people living with HIV and present data from a service evaluation undertaken in the clinic. We conducted an evaluation of the first 52 patients seen in the clinic between 2016 and 2019. We present patient demographic data, assessment outcomes, diagnoses given, and interventions delivered to those seen in the clinic. The average age of attendees was 67. Primary reasons for referral to the clinic included management of complex comorbidities, polypharmacy, and suspected geriatric syndrome (falls, frailty, poor mobility, or cognitive decline). The median (range) number of comorbidities and comedications (non-antiretrovirals) was 7 (2–19) and 9 (1–15), respectively. All attendees had an undetectable viral load. Geriatric syndromes were observed in 26 (50%) patients reviewed in the clinic, with frailty and mental health disease being the most common syndromes. Interventions offered to patients included combination antiretroviral therapy modification, further health investigations, signposting to rehabilitation or social care services, and in-clinic advice. High levels of acceptability among patients and healthcare professionals were reported. The evaluation suggests that specialist geriatric HIV services might play a role in the management of older people with HIV with geriatric syndromes.

Keywords: HIV; geriatrics; comprehensive geriatric assessment

1. Introduction

Increased life expectancy in people living with HIV (PLWH) has brought the challenges of ageing and age-related issues to HIV clinical care [1]. In the UK, 39% of those accessing HIV services are now aged 50 and over, representing over 36,000 individuals considered "older" with HIV [2]. Cohort ageing is set to continue, with modelling work based on PLWH in the Netherlands predicting that, by 2030, 73% will be aged over 50 [3]. Importantly, as PLWH grow older, they appear to be experiencing disproportionally more age-related comorbidities than age-matched HIV-negative populations [4–6]. This is accompanied by greater polypharmacy, as well as issues of functional and cognitive decline, frailty, and falls [7,8]. These issues may be grouped as "geriatric syndromes", highlighting a role for geriatric/elderly medicine within current HIV care [8–10].

How best to deliver geriatric care to PLWH remains unclear. Some service providers advocate for dedicated HIV-ageing services, and a small number of such services have developed or are developing around the world [11]. Joint HIV/speciality clinics have been effective within other specialties [12,13], therefore opening the door to the possibility of HIV-ageing clinics. However, outside of single-organ specialties, the clinical need and criteria for referral are harder to define. One approach is to clinically assess patients at a set age, such as 50 [14], though with the median age of HIV services users in the UK at 46, demand may be excessively high. An alternative could be the use of frailty or frailty syndromes in a "needs-based approach". Tools to identify patients at risk of frailty using scoring methods are increasingly used internationally and have recently been integrated into UK primary care [15]. In October 2019, the European AIDS Clinical Society (EACS) published the first HIV guidance that advocates for frailty screening in older PLWH.

Frailty represents a reduction in physiological reserve that makes one vulnerable to adverse health outcomes [16]. It is prevalent in PLWH and has been associated with falls, incident multi-morbidity, hospitalisation, and death [17–19]. Frailty may present non-specifically (fatigue, weight loss) or as frailty syndromes such as falls, functional decline, and immobility. Additionally, frailty may contribute to medical complexity (polypharmacy and multi-morbidity) and has been associated with low mood and cognitive decline [20,21]. The recommended approach to the assessment and management of frailty is through Comprehensive Geriatric Assessment (CGA) [22]. Proactive identification of frailty and the introduction of CGA can enable early intervention to help PLWH to remain independent. CGA is a multidimensional, interdisciplinary diagnostic process used to determine the medical, psychosocial, and functional capabilities of older adults. Evidence suggests that CGA-based care can improve functional capacity and reduce the risk of institutionalisation when applied to other chronic conditions such as cancer, renal disease, and cardiovascular disease [23–25].

Older PLWH may face a complicated healthcare landscape [26], with HIV-specific management falling down the list of health priorities in favour of age-related issues, which HIV services may be ill-equipped to deal with due to lack of time, resources, or geriatric expertise.

In order to address the issues facing this ageing cohort, the Silver Clinic was established in the Brighton and Sussex University Hospitals Trust. This multi-disciplinary HIV-ageing clinic utilises a CGA approach to assess and manage age-related problems in PLWH. This paper aims to describe the service and results of an initial service evaluation of the clinic.

2. Methods

The Silver Clinic team consists of an (i) HIV consultant physician, (ii) Geriatrics consultant physician, (iii) HIV nurse specialist, and (iv) HIV pharmacist. The clinic operates monthly within the HIV outpatient (Lawson) unit. Clinic referrals come from any HIV healthcare professional (HCP) involved in the care of the patient. The Silver Clinic team is blinded to the process of referral. Current referral criteria are age (>50 years), presence of complex comorbidities and/or polypharmacy, or geriatric syndromes including frailty, falls, and difficulties with activities of daily living. All patients attending the clinic up until October 2019 were included in this evaluation. No exclusion criteria were applied. As this was a service evaluation, ethical approval was not obtained following assessment by the UK Health Research Authority (http://www.hra-decisiontools.org.uk/research/). Written inform consent was provided for the case study.

2.1. Clinic Process

Before attending, new patients are asked to complete a number of screening questionnaires focussed around physical, functional, mood, and cognitive status. The questionnaires are patient-reported outcome measure (PROM) tools that serve two purposes. Firstly, they help practitioners to identify medical, social, or mental health issues that patients have before they are seen in the clinic. Secondly, they can be used to monitor the impact of the service. Prior to first clinic attendance, a multidisciplinary case-based discussion of each patient is organised. This includes: background and PROM review,

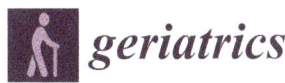

Article

Evaluation of a Combined HIV and Geriatrics Clinic for Older People Living with HIV: The Silver Clinic in Brighton, UK

Tom Levett [1,2], Katie Alford [3], Jonathan Roberts [1], Zoe Adler [1], Juliet Wright [1,4] and Jaime H. Vera [1,3,*]

1. Division of Medicine, Brighton and Sussex University Hospitals NHS Trust, UK; t.levett@nhs.net (T.L.); jonathan.roberts10@nhs.net (J.R.); zoe.adler@nhs.net (Z.A.); juliet.wright6@nhs.net (J.W.)
2. Department of Clinical and Experimental Medicine, Brighton and Sussex Medical School, Falmer, Brighton BN1 9PX, UK
3. Department of Global Health and Infection, Brighton and Sussex Medical School, Falmer, Brighton BN1 9PX, UK; K.Alford2@bsms.ac.uk
4. Department of Medical Education, Brighton and Sussex Medical School, Falmer, Brighton BN1 9PX, UK
* Correspondence: j.vera@bsms.ac.uk

Received: 11 August 2020; Accepted: 13 October 2020; Published: 19 October 2020

Abstract: As life expectancy in people living with HIV (PLWH) has increased, the focus of management has shifted to preventing and treating chronic illnesses, but few services exist for the assessment and management of these individuals. Here, we provide an initial description of a geriatric service for people living with HIV and present data from a service evaluation undertaken in the clinic. We conducted an evaluation of the first 52 patients seen in the clinic between 2016 and 2019. We present patient demographic data, assessment outcomes, diagnoses given, and interventions delivered to those seen in the clinic. The average age of attendees was 67. Primary reasons for referral to the clinic included management of complex comorbidities, polypharmacy, and suspected geriatric syndrome (falls, frailty, poor mobility, or cognitive decline). The median (range) number of comorbidities and comedications (non-antiretrovirals) was 7 (2–19) and 9 (1–15), respectively. All attendees had an undetectable viral load. Geriatric syndromes were observed in 26 (50%) patients reviewed in the clinic, with frailty and mental health disease being the most common syndromes. Interventions offered to patients included combination antiretroviral therapy modification, further health investigations, signposting to rehabilitation or social care services, and in-clinic advice. High levels of acceptability among patients and healthcare professionals were reported. The evaluation suggests that specialist geriatric HIV services might play a role in the management of older people with HIV with geriatric syndromes.

Keywords: HIV; geriatrics; comprehensive geriatric assessment

1. Introduction

Increased life expectancy in people living with HIV (PLWH) has brought the challenges of ageing and age-related issues to HIV clinical care [1]. In the UK, 39% of those accessing HIV services are now aged 50 and over, representing over 36,000 individuals considered "older" with HIV [2]. Cohort ageing is set to continue, with modelling work based on PLWH in the Netherlands predicting that, by 2030, 73% will be aged over 50 [3]. Importantly, as PLWH grow older, they appear to be experiencing disproportionally more age-related comorbidities than age-matched HIV-negative populations [4–6]. This is accompanied by greater polypharmacy, as well as issues of functional and cognitive decline, frailty, and falls [7,8]. These issues may be grouped as "geriatric syndromes", highlighting a role for geriatric/elderly medicine within current HIV care [8–10].

How best to deliver geriatric care to PLWH remains unclear. Some service providers advocate for dedicated HIV-ageing services, and a small number of such services have developed or are developing around the world [11]. Joint HIV/speciality clinics have been effective within other specialties [12,13], therefore opening the door to the possibility of HIV-ageing clinics. However, outside of single-organ specialties, the clinical need and criteria for referral are harder to define. One approach is to clinically assess patients at a set age, such as 50 [14], though with the median age of HIV services users in the UK at 46, demand may be excessively high. An alternative could be the use of frailty or frailty syndromes in a "needs-based approach". Tools to identify patients at risk of frailty using scoring methods are increasingly used internationally and have recently been integrated into UK primary care [15]. In October 2019, the European AIDS Clinical Society (EACS) published the first HIV guidance that advocates for frailty screening in older PLWH.

Frailty represents a reduction in physiological reserve that makes one vulnerable to adverse health outcomes [16]. It is prevalent in PLWH and has been associated with falls, incident multi-morbidity, hospitalisation, and death [17–19]. Frailty may present non-specifically (fatigue, weight loss) or as frailty syndromes such as falls, functional decline, and immobility. Additionally, frailty may contribute to medical complexity (polypharmacy and multi-morbidity) and has been associated with low mood and cognitive decline [20,21]. The recommended approach to the assessment and management of frailty is through Comprehensive Geriatric Assessment (CGA) [22]. Proactive identification of frailty and the introduction of CGA can enable early intervention to help PLWH to remain independent. CGA is a multidimensional, interdisciplinary diagnostic process used to determine the medical, psychosocial, and functional capabilities of older adults. Evidence suggests that CGA-based care can improve functional capacity and reduce the risk of institutionalisation when applied to other chronic conditions such as cancer, renal disease, and cardiovascular disease [23–25].

Older PLWH may face a complicated healthcare landscape [26], with HIV-specific management falling down the list of health priorities in favour of age-related issues, which HIV services may be ill-equipped to deal with due to lack of time, resources, or geriatric expertise.

In order to address the issues facing this ageing cohort, the Silver Clinic was established in the Brighton and Sussex University Hospitals Trust. This multi-disciplinary HIV-ageing clinic utilises a CGA approach to assess and manage age-related problems in PLWH. This paper aims to describe the service and results of an initial service evaluation of the clinic.

2. Methods

The Silver Clinic team consists of an (i) HIV consultant physician, (ii) Geriatrics consultant physician, (iii) HIV nurse specialist, and (iv) HIV pharmacist. The clinic operates monthly within the HIV outpatient (Lawson) unit. Clinic referrals come from any HIV healthcare professional (HCP) involved in the care of the patient. The Silver Clinic team is blinded to the process of referral. Current referral criteria are age (>50 years), presence of complex comorbidities and/or polypharmacy, or geriatric syndromes including frailty, falls, and difficulties with activities of daily living. All patients attending the clinic up until October 2019 were included in this evaluation. No exclusion criteria were applied. As this was a service evaluation, ethical approval was not obtained following assessment by the UK Health Research Authority (http://www.hra-decisiontools.org.uk/research/). Written inform consent was provided for the case study.

2.1. Clinic Process

Before attending, new patients are asked to complete a number of screening questionnaires focussed around physical, functional, mood, and cognitive status. The questionnaires are patient-reported outcome measure (PROM) tools that serve two purposes. Firstly, they help practitioners to identify medical, social, or mental health issues that patients have before they are seen in the clinic. Secondly, they can be used to monitor the impact of the service. Prior to first clinic attendance, a multidisciplinary case-based discussion of each patient is organised. This includes: background and PROM review, evaluation of current clinical problems, and anticipated need of further investigations. All patients then receive a dual consultation with the HIV and elderly medicine physician focused on CGA. This explores patient demographics; social characteristics; comorbidity (including medications); functional, physical, mental health, and frailty status (Table 1). All assessments are triangulated by the multidisciplinary (MDT) to generate a comprehensive individualised management plan that is overseen by the Silver Clinic team and communicated to the referring clinician and the GP where the patient consents. The clinic process for the service is shown in Figure 1.

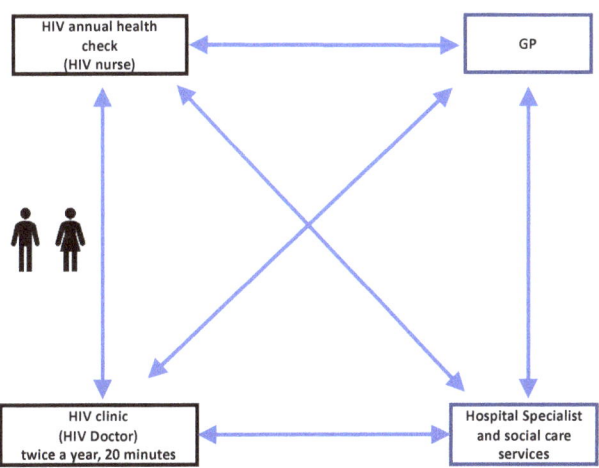

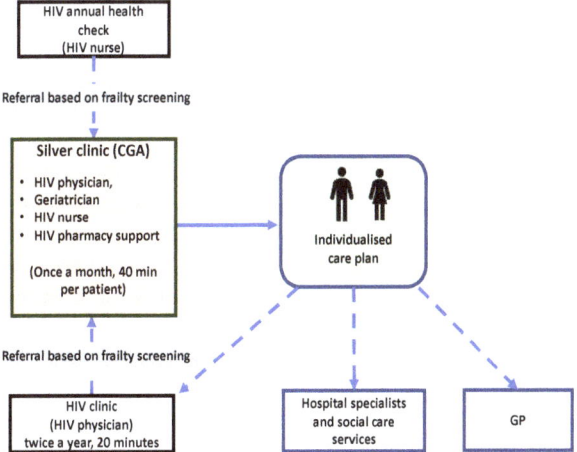

Figure 1. Silver Clinic process and position alongside standard care.

Table 1. Clinical assessments performed within the Silver Clinic.

Test Category	
Blood Tests	Calcium, TFTs, PSA, HbA1c, B12/Folate, Vitamin D
HIV clinical data	Year of diagnosis, nadir and current CD4 cell count, current CD8 cell count, CD4:CD8 ratio, antiretroviral history
Other clinical data	Urinalysis, height, weight, body mass index, blood pressure (lying and standing)
Mood assessment	Hospital Anxiety and Depression Scale
Frailty assessment	FRAIL scale
Patient reported outcome measures	Euroqol-5D-5L Older Peoples' Quality of Life Questionnaire

TFTs, thyroid function tests; PSA, prostate-specific antigens; HbA1c, Haemoglobin A1c.

2.2. Clinical Assessments

Clinical data are drawn from patient notes and most recent routine HIV health checks. Baseline observations, including postural blood pressure and body mass index (BMI), are performed. Blood tests are taken to exclude issues contributing to age-related comorbidities, including vitamin B12 and folate deficiency, associated with neuropsychiatric issues, depression, and demyelinating myelopathy; calcium and 25-OH-Vitamin-D for bone health, falls, and mobility. The full assessment strategy is shown in Error! Reference source not found.

Mood symptoms are assessed using the Hospital Anxiety and Depression Scale (HADS), a short, self-report screening questionnaire for generalised anxiety and depression among patients in non-psychiatric settings. The questionnaire is split into two sub-scales for anxiety (HADS-A) and depression (HADS-D), in which a score ≥11 is considered diagnostic [27].

Patient-reported outcome measures (PROM) include the Older Peoples' Quality of Life Questionnaire (OPQL-brief), a 13-item validated tool for assessing quality of life (QoL) in older people. Scores range from 13 to 65, indicating lowest to highest QoL [28,29]. EuroQol five-dimension descriptive system (EQ-5D-5L) is a brief self-reported measure of generic health and perceived health status that has been used across a number of health conditions and populations [30,31]. The tool includes a visual analogue scale on which individuals indicate their current health state in relation to best and worst imaginable health (100–0, respectively). FRAIL Scale is a clinical screening tool for the identification of frailty. It comprises five self-reported components of fatigue—resistance, ambulation, illnesses, and weight loss—which are scored as present or absent, resulting in a score from 0 to 5. Those scoring 0 are robust, 1–2 prefrail and ≥3 frail [32].

Changes in scores for EQ-5D-5L and OPQL-brief and FRAIL scale at baseline (first assessment) and discharge (12 months) were calculated.

2.3. Patient and Healthcare Professional Satisfaction

A voluntary self-completed survey was completed by patients after the clinic appointment. The survey asked patients to provide qualitative "free-text" feedback of the service, including whether and how it benefitted them and suggestions for service improvement.

An 8-question online questionnaire for healthcare professionals, excluding those working in the Silver Clinic, was accessible from January to March 2018. This was created and hosted using Bristol Online Surveys and distributed via email to all HIV staff. Job role, clinic awareness and referral experience, perceived importance of the clinic, and improvement to older PLWH care were assessed. Partially completed questionnaires were omitted from analysis.

2.4. Statistical Analysis

Descriptive statistics using frequency, mean, or median with respective corresponding percentages, standard deviation, and interquartile range were used to summarize the data. Paired sample *t*-tests were used to evaluate the impact of the Silver Clinic intervention on scores for each PROM (EQ-5D-5L and OPQL-brief and FRAIL scale) from baseline to discharge from the clinic. A framework method of analysis was employed for qualitative data, with frequencies and percentages reported for qualitative variables where grouping was possible [33].

3. Results

From January 2015 to October 2019, the Silver clinic assessed 52 patients. Demographic characteristics, HIV, and other clinical data of clinic attendees are presented in Table 2. The median (range) age of attendees was 67 years (53–87), and the majority were white males identifying as men that have sex with men (MSM), reflecting the clinic population. Attendees had well-controlled chronic HIV, with 100% virally suppressed. Primary referral reason for patients attending the clinic was 67% (35) multimorbidity optimisation, 13% (7) problematic polypharmacy, and 17% (10) suspected geriatric syndrome (falls, frailty, mobility issues, cognitive decline).

Table 2. Summary of patient characteristics.

Clinical Characteristics (*n* = 52)	Median (IQR) Otherwise Stated
Age (years)	67 (53–87)
Male, *n* (%)	47 (90)
White ethnicity, *n* (%)	50 (96)
Identified sexuality, *n* (%)	
MSM	41 (78)
Heterosexual	9 (17)
Other	2 (4)
Current smoker, *n* (%)	17 (32)
Alcohol use, *n* (%)	
Less than 10 units per week	41 (77)
Between 10 and 20 units per week	5 (9)
>20 units per week	3 (4)
Recreational drug use *n* (%)	6 (11)
Comorbidities	7 (2–19)
Comedications	9 (1–15)
QRISK3 *	25 (6–52)
Bone densitometry, *n* (%)	
Osteoporosis	15 (28)
Osteopenia	33 (63)
Normal BMD	4 (7)
HIV Clinical Parameters	
Time since HIV diagnosis: years (median; range)	17 (6–34)
Duration of cART: years (median; range)	17 (5–30)
cART-based regimen *n* (%)	
Protease inhibitor	28 (53)
NNRTI	12 (23)
INSTI	12 (23)
HIV RNA < 50 copies/mL, *n* (%)	52 (100)
Nadir CD4 (cells/µL)	287 (223)
Current CD4 (cells/µL)	563 (368)
CD4:CD8 ratio	0.60 (0.1)

MSM, men who have sex with men; cART, antiretroviral therapy; QRISK®3-2018 cardiovascular risk calculator.

Geriatric syndromes were observed in all patients reviewed in the clinic, with frailty and mental health disease being the most common syndromes, as shown in Figure 2. Patients had a median (IQR) of 7 (2–19) comorbidities. Cardiovascular disease was the most common, reported by 36 patients (70%), followed by neurological disorder (63%), chronic pain syndrome (44%), and mental health conditions (42%). Polypharmacy defined as more than five non-antiretroviral drugs was common, with a median of nine (1–15) medications in addition to their ARVs. The most common comedications at first assessment were cardiovascular medications, followed by analgesics (61%), mental health drugs (40%), and supplements such as vitamins, etc. (53%). Notably, 30% were taking opioid medications for pain and 19% taking benzodiazepines to manage insomnia.

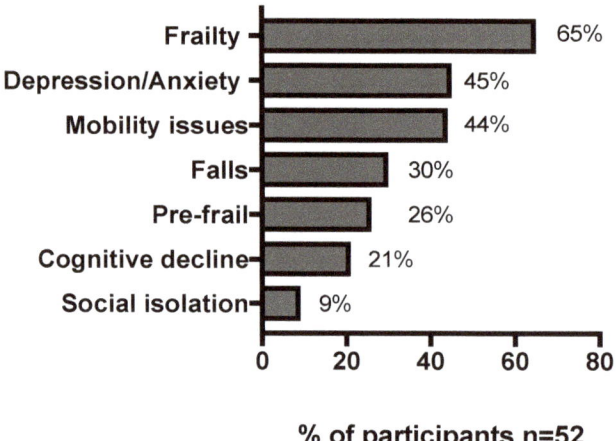

Figure 2. Frequencies of geriatric syndromes.

3.1. Patient-Reported Outcomes

Perceived health-related QoL at first assessment was poor on both the EQ-5D-5L and OPQOL, with mean scores (SD) for the visual scale on the EQ-5D-5L 56.76 (21.2) and 32.76 (8.48) for the OPQOL, respectively. Thirty-four (65%) patients were classified as frail; 14 (26%) were deemed prefrail and 4 (4%) robust using the FRAIL scale. Mental health was assessed using the HADS: 46% (23) had depression or anxiety symptoms at first assessment. No significant changes in EQ-5D-5L and OPQOL-Brief scores were observed at discharge compared to baseline ($p = 0.885$ and $p = 0.218$, respectively). Moreover, no changes in frailty status were observed at discharge using the FRAIL scale ($p = 0.495$)

3.2. Clinic Outcomes

At the point of data analysis, most patients had attended the clinic at least twice, with the median number of visits being two (2–8). The greatest number of visits was eight (two patients). ARV switch recommendations were made in six patients due to toxicities or drug–drug interactions (DDI). Twenty-seven specialist referrals were made, including to the broader multidisciplinary team including physiotherapy and occupational therapy. The clinic has now discharged 42 patients, 4 await follow-up appointment and 6 patients remain open to the service "as needed.

Case Study

To better understand that type of patients we see in the service we described the case of Mr X, a 69-year-old male who was diagnosed with HIV in 1999. He attended the Silver Clinic with complaints of feeling "fed up" and intermittent faecal incontinence. He has multiple comorbidities with associated polypharmacy, as shown in Table 3. He is an ex-smoker who drinks less than 4 units/week, with no recreational drug use. He lives alone and reports feeling socially isolated. He has poor mobility but dislikes using a recommended walking stick and reports three falls during the last 3 months. He relies heavily on his car as he lives in a rural village. His social benefits were reduced last year. His HIV is well controlled, with a current CD4 count of 750 cell/mL and undetectable viral load on a regimen of Darunavir, Ritonavir, and Lamivudine (3TC). His Q-Risk score was 16.5%.

Table 3. Mr X comorbidities and medications.

Medical Comorbidities	Comedications
Type 2 diabetes	1. Paroxetine 40 mg daily
Depression	2. Gabapentin 400 mg twice daily
Osteopenia	3. Aspirin 75 mg daily
Dyslipidaemia	4. Zopiclone 7.5 mg at night
Chronic back pain secondary to (degenerative disease and C-spine injury)	5. Pravastatin 10 mg at night
	6. Zomorph MR 60 mg twice daily
Peripheral neuropathy (ART-related)	7. Metformin 1 g twice daily
Chronic inflammatory demyelinating polyneuropathy unresponsive to immunoglobulin	8. Folic Acid 5 mg daily
	9. Oramorph 5–10 mg as needed

1. Proactive treatment of constipation (causing overflow incontinence) and opioid reduction.
2. Fall prevention through occupational and physiotherapy referral and bone scan with subsequent osteoporosis treatment to reduce fracture risk.
3. Medicines rationalisation with ART modification to a one tablet regimen (Rezolsta: Darunavir/Cobistat), which in turn allowed Zopiclone withdrawal.
4. Signposting to community peer services aimed at increasing socialisation and an application for a disabled parking "Blue Badge" was supported.
5. Referral to Cognitive Behavioural Therapy with the hope that improvements in mental health may also stem from comorbidity optimisation.

At follow-up, despite subjectively his symptoms persisting, QOL based on the EQ-5D-5L and OPQOL had improved.

3.3. Patient Satisfaction

All patients were asked to provide their views of the clinic. Fourteen responses (35%) were received, with 13 (93%) stating that they were "very satisfied" with the service they received, and one respondent was "somewhat satisfied". Qualitative feedback themes identified among respondents were "friendliness/kindness" (28%), "felt listened to" (14%), professional/helpful service (43%). Additional comments referred to the opportunity for in-depth explanation and care coordination.

3.4. Healthcare Professionals' Views of the Silver Clinic

Fourteen (63%) staff responded to our invitation to provide views on the clinic; this included six (43%) doctors, six (43%) nurses, and two (14%) pharmacists. All participants were aware of the clinic, and six (42%) had made referrals. Twelve (85%) believed the Silver Clinic was "very important" for the management of older PLWH and the other two (14%) believed it was "quite important". All respondents felt that the clinic improved the management of older PLWH.

4. Discussion

HIV services have a history of being proactive in their innovation of care models to address the changing needs of their patients. Clear trajectories towards HIV cohort ageing exists in the UK with accompanying age-related medical and psychosocial issues [34]. The Silver Clinic was created to address this emerging need—by employing multidisciplinary working and principles of geriatric care, it has sought to improve the care management of this complex cohort. This service evaluation demonstrates that the average age of Silver Clinic attendees was 67 years old, with the majority referred for management of multimorbidity, polypharmacy, and geriatric/frailty syndromes, which one might anticipate within general elderly medical services.

Classical geriatric syndromes have been demonstrated in older adults, with HIV at higher frequency and earlier age than one might expect for the general population. In one US study of 155 PLWH, median age 57, the prevalence of falls was 26%, and 54% described two or more geriatric syndromes, which were associated with greater comorbidity and lower nadir CD4 count [8]. In our clinic, cohort geriatric syndromes were common, with 44% complaining of mobility issues and 30% experiencing falls. These may be linked to other observed findings of mood disorder in 45% and social isolation in 9%. Social isolation was shown to be more common in older adults with HIV compared to those without (59% vs. 51%, $p < 0.001$) in the Veterans Aging Cohort Study and was associated with increased hospitalisation and mortality [35].

The majority of clinic attendees were frail (65%) based on the FRAIL scale, with a further 26% deemed prefrail. This is considerably higher than frailty prevalence seen in previous studies of PLWH, where frailty based on the Fried Phenotype (FP) ranged from 3 to 28% [36]; using this same measure, prevalence was 3% for frailty and 38% prefrailty in a large UK community study of adults aged 37–73 years [37]. The larger proportion with frailty in our group is reflective of the service model and its remit as a needs-based service, with frailty syndromes within the referral criteria. Targeting of frail and prefrail individuals is vital, however, as both are associated with an increased risk of incident disability in both personal and instrumental activities of daily living and mortality compared to robust individuals [32,38]. Though the natural trajectory of frailty is progressive, studies have demonstrated stability in frail state at one year, as was demonstrated in this non-interventional evaluation of the service [39]. The ongoing presence of frailty in this selected cohort suggests that they may have the most to gain from ongoing geriatric medical input.

The clinic users had a high burden of comorbidity and polypharmacy, particularly mood disorder (45%) and chronic pain, with 30% on regular opiates. High levels of comorbidity and polypharmacy have been noted in cohorts of PLWH [14,40], with both related to greater duration of HIV rather than older age [40]. Chronic opiate use for non-cancer pain is higher in PLWH and is associated with greater comorbidity, and it is an independent risk factor for falls, along with other medications such as benzodiazepines, in this group [41,42]. Comorbidity and polypharmacy, including chronic pain, combined with both frailty and broader geriatric syndromes, would support a multimorbidity-based approach as advocated by the National Institute of Health and Care Excellence. The use of patient-centred care focused around how one's comorbidities and their treatments impact on quality of life and how they align with their life priorities, emphasising strong care coordination [43]. These models are compatible with geriatric principles of care that have been advocated within the HIV literature [11,44,45]. Patient-reported QoL was poor at baseline, with no significant change at one year. This likely reflects the level of comorbidity and functional limitation, alongside unmeasured psychosocial factors [46]. Whilst the former were addressed from a diagnostic perspective, service users could benefit from broader MDT intervention, care coordination, and community-based intervention centred on social prescribing and peer support [47].

It was gratifying to see that the survey of HCPs indicated appropriate awareness of the Silver Clinic, with many reporting the positive improvement to the management of older PLWH as a consequence of the clinic. However, a recent UK survey identified the existence of only two dedicated HIV-ageing services nationwide, with two-thirds of respondents citing insufficient population as the reason for no perceived need for such a service [48], yet we know that a predominantly older adult HIV population is predicted in the near future [3]. HIV-ageing services are now being reported more widely, mainly in high income settings, which are either based on geriatric syndromes or metabolic comorbidities in PLWH [49]. Attendees reported high levels of satisfaction with the clinic, though it should be noted that the number providing feedback was self-selecting and small (35%). However, service user feedback is vital in both the development and evaluation of any new ageing services, with respondents in one survey favouring the maintenance of care within HIV settings, alongside enhanced communication and care coordination [50].

To our knowledge, this represents the first evaluation of a UK-based joint HIV-ageing service run on a needs- rather than age-based approach that utilises CGA principles. It is limited in its presentation of single-site data that are purely descriptive in nature. Other limitations include the small sample size, which also limits the generalizability and reproducibility of the data. Data presented here are not able to define the longer-term benefit regarding preservation of function, admission avoidance, and mortality, as well as the cost-effectiveness of attending the Silver Clinic. However, this is the case for many new services, which are not, at present, being driven by a supporting evidence base. The role of such a clinic, and in particular the role of CGA applied to individuals living with HIV, represents areas of research need within HIV and ageing, which is supported by a nationwide service evaluation on HIV-ageing services that identified a lack of evidence base as a barrier for service development [48]. However, the Silver Clinic is a trail-blazer for other services, with a model that, since conception, meets the recommendations from both the 2019 EACS guidance on frailty screening in PLWH [51] and the 2018 British HIV Association Standards of Care document, which advocates the involvement of a geriatrician with HIV knowledge in the care of service users requiring complex HIV care [52].

5. Conclusions

We have operationalised a dedicated HIV-ageing service founded on geriatric medicine principles that is acceptable to both service users and referrers within HIV medicine. Referral pathways have identified a clinic cohort with high burden of frailty, comorbidity, and geriatric syndromes that might benefit from comprehensive geriatric assessment. Ongoing evaluation and research in this area is crucial to demonstrate the effectiveness of this model of care and/or help in building an evidence base to support other models of care for those ageing with HIV.

Author Contributions: J.H.V., K.A., J.W. and T.L. contributed to the study concept and design, analysis and interpretation of data and drafting of manuscript. J.R., Z.A., contributed to the acquisition of data and revision of the manuscript. All authors have read and agreed to the published version of the manuscript.

Funding: This work was supported by Brighton and Sussex Medical School. Grant code: G25342.

Conflicts of Interest: J.H.V. has received travel and research grants from and has been speaker/advisor for Merck, Janssen Cilag, Piramal, ViiV Healthcare, and Gilead Sciences. J.W. and T.L. have received travel and being speakers for Gilead. J.R. and Z.A. have no disclosures.

References

1. Harris, T.G.; Rabkin, M.; El-Sadr, W.M. Achieving the fourth 90. *AIDS* **2018**, *32*, 1563–1569. [CrossRef] [PubMed]
2. Nash, S.; Desai, S.; Croxford, S.; Guerra, L.; Lowndes, C.; Connor, N.; Gill, O.N. *Progress towards Ending the HIV Epidemic in the United Kingdom: 2018 Report*; Public Health England: London, UK, 2018.
3. Smit, M.; Brinkman, K.; Geerlings, S.; Smit, C.; Thyagarajan, K.; Van Sighem, A.; De Wolf, F.; Hallett, T.B. Future challenges for clinical care of an ageing population infected with HIV: A modelling study. *Lancet Infect. Dis.* **2015**, *15*, 810–818. [CrossRef]
4. Schouten, J.; Wit, F.W.; Stolte, I.G.; Kootstra, N.A.; Van Der Valk, M.; Geerlings, S.E.; Prins, M.; Reiss, P.; Kooij, K.W.; Van Zoest, R.A.; et al. Cross-sectional comparison of the prevalence of age-associated comorbidities and their risk factors between HIV-infected and uninfected individuals: The AGEhIV cohort study. *Clin. Infect. Dis.* **2014**, *59*, 1787–1797. [CrossRef] [PubMed]
5. Althoff, K.N.; Jacobson, L.P.; Cranston, R.D.; Detels, R.; Phair, J.P.; Li, X.; Margolick, J.B.; for the Multicenter AIDS cohort study (MACS). Age, comorbidities, and AIDS predict a frailty phenotype in men who have sex with men. *J. Gerontol. Ser. A Biol. Sci. Med. Sci.* **2013**, *69*, 189–198. [CrossRef]
6. Guaraldi, G.; Orlando, G.; Zona, S.; Menozzi, M.; Carli, F.; Garlassi, E.; Berti, A.; Rossi, E.; Roverato, A.; Palella, F. Premature age-related comorbidities among HIV-infected persons compared with the general population. *Clin. Infect. Dis.* **2011**, *53*, 1120–1126. [CrossRef] [PubMed]

7. Halloran, M.; Boyle, C.; Kehoe, B.; Bagkeris, E.; Mallon, P.; A Post, F.; Vera, J.; Williams, I.; Anderson, J.; Winston, A.; et al. Polypharmacy and drug–drug interactions in older and younger people living with HIV: The POPPY study. *Antivir. Ther.* **2019**, *24*, 193–201. [CrossRef]
8. Greene, M.; Covinsky, K.E.; Valcour, V.; Miao, Y.; Madamba, J.; Lampiris, H.; Cenzer, I.S.; Martin, J.; Deeks, S.G. Geriatric syndromes in older HIV-infected adults. *J. Acquir. Immune Defic. Syndr.* **2015**, *69*, 161–167. [CrossRef] [PubMed]
9. Guaraldi, G.; Rockwood, K. Geriatric-HIV medicine is born. *Clin. Infect. Dis.* **2017**, *65*, 507–509. [CrossRef] [PubMed]
10. Hawkins, K.L.; Brown, T.T.; Margolick, J.B.; Erlandson, K.M. Geriatric syndromes: New frontiers in HIV and sarcopenia. *AIDS* **2017**, *31*, S137–S146. [CrossRef]
11. Singh, H.K.; Del Carmen, T.; Freeman, R.; Glesby, M.J.; Siegler, E.L. From one syndrome to many: Incorporating geriatric consultation into HIV care. *Clin. Infect. Dis.* **2017**, *65*, 501–506. [CrossRef]
12. McClure, M.; Singh, G.J.; Rayment, M.; Jones, R.; Levy, J.B. Clinical outcomes of a combined HIV and renal clinic. *Clin. Kidney J.* **2012**, *5*, 530–534. [CrossRef] [PubMed]
13. Koganti, S.; Loes, S.K.-D.; Hutchinson, S.; Johnson, M.; Rakhit, R.D. Management of cardiovascular conditions in a cohort of patients with HIV: Experience from a joint HIV/cardiology clinic. *Clin. Med.* **2015**, *15*, 442–446. [CrossRef] [PubMed]
14. Waters, L.; Patterson, B.; Scourfield, A.; Hughes, A.; De Silva, S.; Gazzard, B.; Barton, S.; Asboe, D.; Pozniak, A.; Boffito, M. A dedicated clinic for HIV-positive individuals over 50 years of age: A multidisciplinary experience. *Int. J. STD AIDS* **2012**, *23*, 546–552. [CrossRef]
15. NHS England; LTC Team. *Toolkit for General Practice in Supporting Older People Living with Frailty*; NHS England: London, UK, 2017.
16. Clegg, A.; Young, J.; Iliffe, S.; Rikkert, M.O.; Rockwood, K. Frailty in elderly people. *Lancet* **2013**, *381*, 752–762. [CrossRef]
17. Tassiopoulos, K.; Abdo, M.; Wu, K.; Koletar, S.L.; Palella, F.J.; Kalayjian, R.; Taiwo, B.; Erlandson, K.M. Frailty is strongly associated with increased risk of recurrent falls among older HIV-infected adults. *AIDS* **2017**, *31*, 2287–2294. [CrossRef]
18. Guaraldi, G.; Brothers, T.D.; Zona, S.; Stentarelli, C.; Carli, F.; Malagoli, A.; Santoro, A.; Menozzi, M.; Mussi, C.; Mussini, C.; et al. A frailty index predicts survival and incident multimorbidity independent of markers of HIV disease severity. *AIDS* **2015**, *29*, 1633–1641. [CrossRef] [PubMed]
19. Akgun, K.M.; Tate, J.P.; Crothers, K.; Crystal, S.; Leaf, D.A.; Womack, J.; Brown, T.T.; Justice, A.C.; Oursler, K.K. An adapted frailty-related phenotype and the VACS index as predictors of hospitalization and mortality in HIV-infected and uninfected individuals. *J. Acquir. Immune Defic. Syndr.* **2014**, *67*, 397–404. [CrossRef]
20. Collard, R.M.; Comijs, H.C.; Naarding, P.; Penninx, B.W.; Milaneschi, Y.; Ferrucci, L.; Voshaar, R.C.O. Frailty as a predictor of the incidence and course of depressed mood. *J. Am. Med. Dir. Assoc.* **2015**, *16*, 509–514. [CrossRef]
21. Underwood, J.; Robertson, K.R.; Winston, A. Could antiretroviral neurotoxicity play a role in the pathogenesis of cognitive impairment in treated HIV disease? *AIDS* **2015**, *29*, 253–261. [CrossRef]
22. British Geriatric Society, Fit for Frailty. 2017. Available online: https://www.bgs.org.uk/sites/default/files/content/resources/files/2018-05-14/fff2_short.pdf (accessed on 1 June 2019).
23. Ellis, G.; Gardner, M.; Tsiachristas, A.; Langhorne, P.; Burke, O.; Harwood, R.H.; Conroy, S.P.; Kircher, T.; Somme, D.; Saltvedt, I.; et al. Comprehensive geriatric assessment for older adults admitted to hospital. *Cochrane Database Syst. Rev.* 2017. [CrossRef]
24. Stuck, A.E.; Iliffe, S. Comprehensive geriatric assessment for older adults. *BMJ* **2011**, *343*, d6799. [CrossRef]
25. Garrard, J.W.; Cox, N.J.; Dodds, R.M.; Roberts, H.C.; Sayer, A.A. Comprehensive geriatric assessment in primary care: A systematic review. *Aging Clin. Exp. Res.* **2019**, *32*, 197–205. [CrossRef] [PubMed]
26. Terrence Higgins Trust, Uncharted Territory: A Report into the First Generation Growing Older with HIV. 2017. Available online: https://www.tht.org.uk/sites/default/files/2018-03/uncharted_territory_final_low-res.pdf (accessed on 13 October 2020).
27. Zigmond, A.S.; Snaith, R.P. The hospital anxiety and depression scale. *Acta Psychiatr. Scand.* **1983**, *67*, 361–370. [CrossRef] [PubMed]

28. Bowling, A.; Hankins, M.; Windle, G.; Bilotta, C.; Grant, R. A short measure of quality of life in older age: The performance of the brief older people's quality of life questionnaire (OPQOL-brief). *Arch. Gerontol. Geriatr.* **2013**, *56*, 181–187. [CrossRef]
29. Kaambwa, B.; Gill, L.; McCaffrey, N.; Lancsar, E.; Cameron, I.D.; Crotty, M.; Gray, L.; Ratcliffe, J. An empirical comparison of the OPQoL-Brief, EQ-5D-3 L and ASCOT in a community dwelling population of older people. *Health Qual. Life Outcomes* **2015**, *13*, 164. [CrossRef] [PubMed]
30. Herdman, M.; Gudex, C.; Lloyd, A.; Janssen, M.; Kind, P.; Parkin, D.; Bonsel, G.; Badia, X. Development and preliminary testing of the new five-level version of EQ-5D (EQ-5D-5L). *Qual. Life Res.* **2011**, *20*, 1727–1736. [CrossRef]
31. Dyer, M.T.D.; A Goldsmith, K.; Sharples, L.S.; Buxton, M.J. A review of health utilities using the EQ-5D in studies of cardiovascular disease. *Health Qual. Life Outcomes* **2010**, *8*, 13. [CrossRef]
32. Kojima, G. Quick and Simple FRAIL Scale predicts incident activities of daily living (ADL) and instrumental ADL (IADL) disabilities: A systematic review and meta-analysis. *J. Am. Med. Dir. Assoc.* **2018**, *19*, 1063–1068. [CrossRef]
33. Gale, N.K.; Heath, G.; Cameron, E.; Rashid, S.; Redwood, S. Using the framework method for the analysis of qualitative data in multi-disciplinary health research. *BMC Med. Res. Methodol.* **2013**, *13*, 117. [CrossRef]
34. Bagkeris, E.; Burgess, L.; Mallon, P.W.; Post, F.A.; Boffito, M.; Sachikonye, M.; Anderson, J.; Asboe, D.; Garvey, L.; Vera, J.; et al. Cohort profile: The Pharmacokinetic and clinical observations in PeoPle over fiftY (POPPY) study. *Int. J. Epidemiol.* **2018**, *47*, 1391–1392e. [CrossRef]
35. Greysen, S.R.; Horwitz, L.I.; Covinsky, K.E.; Gordon, K.; Ohl, M.; Justice, A.C. Does social isolation predict hospitalization and mortality among HIV+ and uninfected older veterans? *J. Am. Geriatr. Soc.* **2013**, *61*, 1456–1463. [CrossRef] [PubMed]
36. Levett, T.J.; Cresswell, F.V.; Malik, M.A.; Fisher, M.; Wright, J. Systematic Review of Prevalence and predictors of frailty in individuals with human immunodeficiency virus. *J. Am. Geriatr. Soc.* **2016**, *64*, 1006–1014. [CrossRef] [PubMed]
37. Hanlon, P.; I Nicholl, B.; Jani, B.D.; Lee, D.; McQueenie, R.; Mair, F.S. Frailty and pre-frailty in middle-aged and older adults and its association with multimorbidity and mortality: A prospective analysis of 493 737 UK Biobank participants. *Lancet Public Health* **2018**, *3*, e323–e332. [CrossRef]
38. Kojima, G. Frailty Defined by FRAIL Scale as a predictor of mortality: A systematic review and meta-analysis. *J. Am. Med. Dir. Assoc.* **2018**, *19*, 480–483. [CrossRef]
39. Gill, T.M.; Gahbauer, E.A.; Allore, H.G.; Han, L. Transitions between frailty states among community-living older persons. *Arch. Intern. Med.* **2006**, *166*, 418–423. [CrossRef] [PubMed]
40. Guaraldi, G.; Malagoli, A.; Calcagno, A.; Mussi, C.; Celesia, B.M.; Carli, F.; Piconi, S.; De Socio, G.V.; Cattelan, A.M.; Orofino, G.; et al. The increasing burden and complexity of multi-morbidity and polypharmacy in geriatric HIV patients: A cross sectional study of people aged 65–74 years and more than 75 years. *BMC Geriatr.* **2018**, *18*, 99. [CrossRef]
41. Silverberg, M.J.; Ray, G.T.; Saunders, K.; Rutter, C.M.; Campbell, C.I.; Merrill, J.O.; Sullivan, M.D.; Banta-Green, C.J.; Von Korff, M.; Weisner, C. Prescription long-term opioid use in HIV-infected patients. *Clin. J. Pain* **2012**, *28*, 39–46. [CrossRef]
42. Erlandson, K.M.; Allshouse, A.A.; Jankowski, C.M.; Duong, S.; Mawhinney, S.; Kohrt, W.M.; Campbell, T.B. Risk factors for falls in HIV-infected persons. *J. Acquir. Immune Defic. Syndr.* **2012**, *61*, 484–489. [CrossRef]
43. NICE, Multimorbidity: Clinical Assessment and Management. National Institute of Health Research Guidelines. 2016. Available online: https://www.nice.org.uk/guidance/ng56 (accessed on 13 October 2020).
44. Greene, M.; Justice, A.C.; Covinsky, K.E. Assessment of geriatric syndromes and physical function in people living with HIV. *Virulence* **2016**, *8*, 586–598. [CrossRef] [PubMed]
45. Levett, T.; Wright, J. How to assess and manage frailty in patients with HIV. *Sex. Transm. Infect.* **2017**, *93*, 476–477. [CrossRef] [PubMed]
46. Langebeek, N.; Kooij, K.W.; Wit, F.W.; Stolte, I.G.; Sprangers, M.A.G.; Reiss, P.; Nieuwkerk, P.T. Impact of comorbidity and ageing on health-related quality of life in HIV-positive and HIV-negative individuals. *AIDS* **2017**, *31*, 1471–1481. [CrossRef] [PubMed]
47. Vargas, R.B.; Cunningham, W.E. Evolving trends in medical care-coordination for patients with HIV and AIDS. *Curr. HIV/AIDS Rep.* **2006**, *3*, 149–153. [CrossRef] [PubMed]

48. Cresswell, F.; Levett, T. Specialist care of older adults with HIV infection in the UK: A service evaluation. *HIV Med.* **2017**, *18*, 519–524. [CrossRef] [PubMed]
49. Siegler, E.L.; O Burchett, C.; Glesby, M.J. Older people with HIV are an essential part of the continuum of HIV care. *J. Int. AIDS Soc.* **2018**, *21*, e25188. [CrossRef]
50. Pollard, A.; Llewellyn, C.; Cooper, V.; Sachikonye, M.; Perry, N.; Nixon, E.; Miners, A.; Youssef, E.; Sabin, C. Patients' perspectives on the development of HIV services to accommodate ageing with HIV: A qualitative study. *Int. J. STD AIDS* **2017**, *29*, 483–490. [CrossRef]
51. European AIDS Clinical Society EACS. Available online: https://www.eacsociety.org/files/2019_guidelines-10.0_final.pdf (accessed on 13 October 2020).
52. BHIVA, Standards of Care for People Living with HIV. 2018. Available online: https://www.bhiva.org/file/KrfaFqLZRlBhg/BHIVA-Standards-of-Care-2018.pdf (accessed on 13 October 2020).

Publisher's Note: MDPI stays neutral with regard to jurisdictional claims in published maps and institutional affiliations.

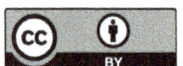

© 2020 by the authors. Licensee MDPI, Basel, Switzerland. This article is an open access article distributed under the terms and conditions of the Creative Commons Attribution (CC BY) license (http://creativecommons.org/licenses/by/4.0/).

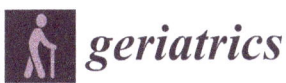

Protocol

Comprehensive Geriatric Assessment for Frail Older People in Swedish Acute Care Settings (CGA-Swed): A Randomised Controlled Study

Katarina Wilhelmson [1,2,3,*], Isabelle Andersson Hammar [1,3], Anna Ehrenberg [4], Johan Niklasson [5], Jeanette Eckerblad [6], Niklas Ekerstad [7,8], Theresa Westgård [1,3], Eva Holmgren [1,3], N. David Åberg [2,9] and Synneve Dahlin Ivanoff [1,3]

1. Department of Health and Rehabilitation, Institute of Neuroscience and Physiology, Sahlgrenska Academy, University of Gothenburg, 405 30 Gothenburg, Sweden; isabelle.a-h@neuro.gu.se (I.A.H.); theresa.westgard@neuro.gu.se (T.W.); eva.holmgren@neuro.gu.se (E.H.); synneve.dahlin-ivanoff@neuro.gu.se (S.D.I.)
2. Region Västra Götaland, Sahlgrenska University Hospital, Department of Acute Medicine and Geriatrics, 413 45 Gothenburg, Sweden; david.aberg@medic.gu.se
3. Centre for Aging and Health—AgeCap, University of Gothenburg, 405 30 Gothenburg, Sweden
4. School of Education, Health and Social Studies, Dalarna University, 791 31 Falun, Sweden; aeh@du.se
5. Department of Community Medicine and Rehabilitation Geriatric Medicine, Sunderby Research Unit, Umeå University, 901 87 Umeå, Sweden; johan.niklasson@umu.se
6. Department of Neurobiology, Care Sciences and Society, Karolinska Institutet, 171 77 Solna, Sweden; jeanette.eckerblad@ki.se
7. Region Department of Medical and Health Sciences, Division of Health Care Analysis, Linköping University, 581 83 Linköping, Sweden; niklas.ekerstad@vgregion.se
8. Department of Research and Development, NU Hospital Group, 461 73 Trollhättan, Sweden
9. Department of Internal Medicine, Institute of Medicine, Sahlgrenska Academy, University of Gothenburg, 405 30 Gothenburg, Sweden
* Correspondence: katarina.wilhelmson@gu.se

Received: 11 December 2019; Accepted: 22 January 2020; Published: 24 January 2020

Abstract: The aim of the study is to evaluate the effects of the Comprehensive Geriatric Assessment (CGA) for frail older people in Swedish acute hospital settings – the CGA-Swed study. In this study protocol, we present the study design, the intervention and the outcome measures as well as the baseline characteristics of the study participants. The study is a randomised controlled trial with an intervention group receiving the CGA and a control group receiving medical assessment without the CGA. Follow-ups were conducted after 1, 6 and 12 months, with dependence in activities of daily living (ADL) as the primary outcome measure. The study group consisted of frail older people (75 years and older) in need of acute medical hospital care. The study design, randomisation and process evaluation carried out were intended to ensure the quality of the study. Baseline data show that the randomisation was successful and that the sample included frail older people with high dependence in ADL and with a high comorbidity. The CGA contributed to early recognition of frail older people's needs and ensured a care plan and follow-up. This study is expected to show positive effects on frail older people's dependence in ADL, life satisfaction and satisfaction with health and social care.

Keywords: frail older people; comprehensive geriatric assessment; activities of daily living; geriatric; hospital care

1. Introduction

Even though health care in Sweden is one of the best worldwide [1], many frail older people do not receive appropriate health care. Today's specialised acute care is poorly adapted to the comprehensive care needs of frail older people and, therefore, exposes them to avoidable risks, such as loss of functional capacities, resulting in unnecessary health and social care needs as well as increased mortality [2]. In addition to appropriate specialised care when needed, assessments that are both comprehensive and person-centred are required to provide satisfactory and appropriate care to older people with complex needs [3]. Frailty is a state of decreased reserve resistance to stressors as a result of cumulative decline across multiple physiological systems, causing vulnerability to different outcomes such as falls, hospitalisation, institutionalisation and mortality [3–5]. Frail older people are at risk of further deterioration if their needs are not acknowledged [3]. The prevalence of frailty increases with age and is associated with an elevated risk of adverse health outcomes. Within Europe, the overall prevalence of frailty for people 65 years and older is approximately 10% with the northern countries having lower prevalence than the southern. Sweden has among the lowest, approximately 5% [6,7].

Previous research has found that the Comprehensive Geriatric Assessment (CGA) in acute hospital care is beneficial for frail older patients [8–11] and might be cost effective [12–14]. The CGA adopts a multi-dimensional team approach for assessing medical, functional, psychosocial and environmental needs [15]. The goal is to identify needs and provide support to help older people to be as independent as possible in their daily living. Key components of CGA interventions include coordinated multi-disciplinary assessment; geriatric medicine competence; identification of medical, physical, social and psychological problems; and the formation of a plan for care including appropriate rehabilitation [10]. Other components associated with improved outcomes of CGA are the ability to directly implement treatment recommendations made by the multi-disciplinary team and long-term follow-up [10]. Another key feature is the identification of frail patients. The acute care of older patients currently often takes place in acute care settings with short lengths of stay [16], and the CGA requires time and staff. For efficient use of healthcare resources, it is therefore important to identify those who can benefit the most from such an assessment by screening for frailty [17]. According to consensus from an international expert group, all persons aged ≥70 years should be screened for frailty [3]. Screening for frailty at the emergency department has proven effective [18,19] for identifying those in need of a more comprehensive assessment.

The benefits of CGA are highlighted in systematic reviews by both the Swedish Agency for Health Technology Assessment and Assessment of Social Services (SBU) and the Cochrane Collaboration [8–11]. Positive effects of CGA for frail older patients have been shown in the form of improved functional status, increased ability to remain in own housing and fewer readmissions. These results are important both for the frail older person and for society at large, because the CGA increases the individual's possibility to live independently in their own home and leads to a decreased need for in-hospital and institutional care. However, both reviews state that substantial knowledge gaps concerning the effects of the CGA remain due to the lack of recent studies as well as those evaluating the CGA using validated measures [8,10,11]. Studies on the CGA have been conducted in various countries with different healthcare systems and demographic profiles. The CGA is a complex intervention that is highly dependent upon the context in which it is used [16], and there are very few recent studies carried out within the Swedish healthcare system thus limiting generalisation to the Swedish context.

Swedish healthcare has undergone dramatic changes over the last decades, resulting in decreased numbers of hospital beds and shorter hospital stays [20], especially evident in geriatric hospital care [21]. This has led to Sweden having the lowest per capita hospital bed rate in Europe [20]. Despite the benefits of the CGA, it is a rather unknown concept within Swedish hospital care [11]. Over the past few years, there has been an increased interest, and many geriatric wards have implemented this way of working. However, geriatric hospital care is unevenly distributed within Sweden with a higher density within the bigger cities and university hospitals [11]. The CGA, within a Swedish community setting, has recently proven successful in maintaining/improving independence in activities of daily living (ADL) [22] as has the CGA in outpatient care [23]. One recent controlled study of an acute CGA unit reported the positive effects on health-related quality of life and mortality without higher costs [24]. Besides these studies, recent studies within Swedish acute care are scarce. Other limitations of these reviews are that many of the studies are dated, have limited sample sizes and have other methodological flaws [8–11]. More knowledge is needed on the implementation, effectiveness and cost effectiveness of the CGA in modern acute care settings. There is also a need to further investigate the relationship between frailty and the CGA as pointed out in a recent umbrella review of the CGA by Parker et al. [25]. This review also states that patient-related outcomes of the CGA—such as health-related quality of life, well-being and participation—are scarcely reported.

Thus, there is still a need for studies on the CGA and interventions using the CGA to improve acute care for frail older people in Swedish health care settings. To meet this need, we designed the study "Comprehensive Geriatric Assessment for Frail Older People in Swedish Acute Care Settings (CGA-Swed): A Randomised Controlled Study" with the purpose of improving hospital care for frail older people by implementing the CGA in Swedish acute care and testing the effects of the CGA in a randomised controlled study (RCT). The intervention was planned and elaborated in collaboration between professionals and researchers. The study includes both quantitative and qualitative analyses of the effects of CGA and a process evaluation of the implementation process throughout the intervention period. It started with a pilot and feasibility study that showed that the intervention—the CGA—and the research procedures were feasible [26]. There were also results indicating that the CGA increased patient safety [26]. Qualitative interviews with frail older people receiving care with the CGA at the intervention ward showed that they felt respected as persons when they were enabled to understand, engage in communication and participate in decisions [27]. The process evaluation alongside the RCT will add to the knowledge on the implementation of the CGA.

Aim and Research Questions

The aim of the study was to evaluate the effects of the CGA for frail older people in Swedish acute hospital settings. The study addresses the following research questions:

Can the Comprehensive Geriatric Assessment for frail older people in Swedish acute hospital settings:

1. Maintain independence in activities of daily living, functional status, health-related quality of life and life satisfaction?
2. Increase satisfaction with health care?
3. Reduce hospital and primary health care consumption?

How feasible and acceptable are the study processes and procedures of the CGA from the perspective of care givers and older persons in Swedish settings?

Ethical approval was obtained for the study, ref. no: 4,899-15, Regional Ethical Review Board in Gothenburg. Trial Registration: ClinicalTrials.gov, NCT02773914.

This paper presents the study design, the intervention, baseline characteristics and the outcome measures of the study in accordance with the recommendations for reporting pragmatic randomised controlled trials by CONSORT [28].

2. Material and Methods

2.1. Project Context

The intervention "Comprehensive Geriatric Assessment for frail older people in Swedish acute care settings" took place at Sahlgrenska University Hospital/Sahlgrenska in Gothenburg, Sweden. Gothenburg is the second largest city in Sweden, situated on the west coast. It had 556,000 inhabitants in the year 2016. Sahlgrenska University Hospital is the regional hospital for Gothenburg and the surrounding municipalities, serving a total of almost one million inhabitants in 2016. The percentage of the population of people aged 75 and over for this region was 7.4% in 2016, compared to 8.6% for all of Sweden [29].

2.2. Study Design

The study was a two-armed randomised controlled trial that started with a pilot study in 2016. The CGA is a complex intervention that influences clinicians' cognitive processes, requires multi-disciplinary collaboration and organisation of healthcare and is highly dependent upon the context in which it is used [16]. An RCT conducted in isolation may not be sufficient to provide guidance for decision makers in healthcare on whether or not to implement research findings. In addition, it is of interest to explore why, for whom and under what circumstances the intervention works. Thus, there was a process evaluation alongside the complex intervention as recommended by the Medical Research Council [30]. The pilot study and the process evaluation provide insight into the function and consequences of the intervention—why it works or fails—and help assess the feasibility of the intervention and research procedures. They also provide data on the number of factors that need to be assessed to successfully monitor and evaluate outcomes. This was an important part of the design that will shed light on real-life conditions that may be challenging in implementing the CGA. The pilot study with the first 30 participants showed that both the intervention and the research procedures worked well [26].

2.3. Study Population

The study group included 155 older people who sought acute medical care at the emergency department during the period between March 2016 and December 2018. Inclusion criteria were that participants were to be ≥75 years of age, in need of acute in-hospital care and screened as frail according to the FRESH-screening instrument. This screening instrument was chosen, since it was already implemented in clinical use, has high sensitivity and specificity (81% and 80%) for screening for frailty in acute settings and has an excellent clinical value [19]. It consists of four questions regarding dependence in shopping, tiredness, fatigue and risk of falling. Two or more "yes" responses indicate frailty. Exclusion criteria were not being screened as frail according to the FRESH-screening instrument, being admitted through a "fast track" for direct admission to a designated ward (for predefined diagnosis such as stroke, acute myocardial infarction and hip fracture) and having an acute severe condition requiring a higher level of care (e.g., intensive care) than the intervention ward. Cognitive impairment was not an exclusion criterion, and if the participant could not give informed consent due to the fact of cognitive impairment ($n = 11$), informed consent was obtained from next of kin.

2.4. Intervention Group

The intervention was the ward working according to the Comprehensive Geriatric Assessment. Key components of the CGA are multi-disciplinary teamwork, use of a person-centred approach [31], comprehensive assessments, treatment and rehabilitation, discharge planning and follow-up (see Figure 1). The multi-disciplinary team consisted of a physician, registered nurse (RN), assistant nurse (AN), physiotherapist (PT) and occupational therapist (OT) as well as other team members, such as a social worker (SW) and dietician, if needed. A pharmacist would have been valuable to include in the team, but this is not common in Swedish hospital wards. The senior physicians at the intervention wards were all specialist in geriatrics. The team had primary and continuing responsibility for assessment, planning of hospital care and discharge. Assessments of medical status, self-assessed health, functional status, psychological status, social situation and environment (see Table 1) were administered to ensure a comprehensive evaluation of the health and life situation of the frail older patient. The team used a person-centred approach [31] to individualise the assessment. A team conference was held every weekday to promote the sharing of information, experiences and competences in order to individualise the care for each patient.

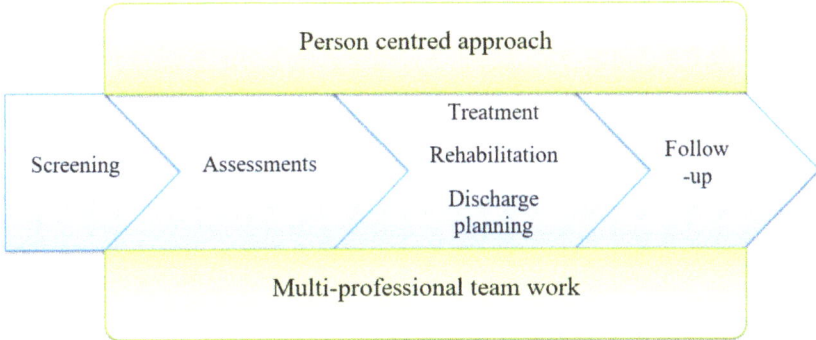

Figure 1. Key components of the Comprehensive Geriatric Assessment (CGA).

The content of the CGA was adapted to local routines and experiences and was elaborated in collaboration between the researchers and those working in the clinical setting where the intervention took place. This was to ensure that the CGA would be both clinically acceptable and evidence based. All personal at the intervention ward received education (i.e., information and workshops) on the CGA prior to the start of the study. During the whole study period, the researchers had meetings with representatives from the different professionals in order to follow how the teams experienced working according to the CGA.

The CGA starts at the intervention ward and continues throughout the hospital stay. It is individualised and unique for each patient, based on the key components in Figure 1 and the assessments in Table 1, providing a comprehensive assessment tailored for each person.

Table 1. Assessments included in the CGA.

Domain	Assessment	Main Professional Responsible
Medical status	Illness burden/medical review	Physician
	Symptoms	Physician/RN
	Somatic status	Physician
	Pharmaceutical review	Physician
	Nutritional status	RN/Dietician
Self-assessed health	Self-assessed health	Physician/RN
Functional status	Activities of daily living	OT
	Physical function	PT
	Sight and hearing	RN/AN
Psychological status	Cognition	OT
	Depression	Physician
Social situation	Social network/informal support	RN/SW
	Formal support	RN/SW
	Financial support	RN/SW
Environment	Living conditions	RN/SW/AN
	Transports	RN/SW/AN
	Accessibility and assistive devices	OT/SW

RN = registered nurse; OT = occupational therapist; PT = physiotherapist; AN = assistant nurse; SW = social worker.

2.5. Control Group

The control group received the usual acute hospital care, i.e., care given at an ordinary medical hospital ward without a specialised multi-disciplinary team approach and without the CGA. The assessments and care provided at the control wards were based on the acute problem/symptom that the patients had and did not include the comprehensive and person-centred approach to the health and life situation of the patient inherent in a CGA. The occupational therapist and the physiotherapist worked more as consultants, and the amount of resources from occupational therapists and physiotherapists were lower at the control wards compared with the intervention wards. At the control ward, they did not perform functional tests, assessments of social network and total disease burden on all frail older patients. The senior physician at the control wards were specialists in internal medicine and were not geriatricians.

2.6. Procedures of the Intervention Study

Older patients who were screened as frail and were in need of in-hospital care were invited to participate in the study during the stay in the Emergency Department (ED). Those who agreed to participate were then randomised into control or intervention groups. Randomisation was done by computer-generated numbers and assigned by one of the researchers using QuickCalcs at GraphPad [32]. The allocation was concealed in numbered opaque envelopes. When a patient consented to participate, the hospital bed coordinator opened the envelope and admitted the patient to the designated ward. The intervention group was admitted to the ward according to the CGA and the control group to a general acute medical ward.

Baseline measures were collected by a research assistant who gathered data from the frail older patient and/or from the medical records during the hospital stay. Six participants were discharged before the baseline interview was completed. For these participants, parts or the whole of the baseline data collection was carried out in the participants' homes as soon as possible after discharge. One participant was discharged to a surgical ward at a different hospital before the baseline interview, suffered a stroke after surgery and, thus, was admitted to the stroke ward at the intervention hospital. For this participant, the baseline interview was conducted retrospectively at the same time as the one-month follow-up which was performed during the stay at the stroke ward.

Follow-up interviews were performed in the older person's home at 1, 6 and 12 months after hospital discharge. The follow-ups were performed using a structured questionnaire including questions about demographic data and assessments of outcome measures. The interviews lasted for approximately 1.5 h. Proxy interviews were done if the participant had a cognitive impairment making them unable to participate in parts or the whole of the baseline/follow-up data collection. No proxy interview was necessary at baseline. However, for a few participants, a next of kin was present during parts of the interview, providing additional information for participants who had difficulties remembering. Next of kin were also present at many follow-up interviews, supplementing the information provided during the interviews. A few of the follow-ups required proxy interviews. Whenever possible, the same person performed all follow-ups for the same participant, minimising the number of people that a frail older participant needed to meet.

The participants could not be blinded to the ward they were being admitted to, but they were not aware at which ward the intervention took place. However, they might have realised if they were administered the CGA. The wards could not be blinded to allocation, because the ward was the allocation. Not all patients at the intervention and control wards were included in the study, and the staff at the wards was not informed which patients were included in the study. In this respect, the staff could be seen as blinded. However, they might have observed the research assistant performing the baseline data collection and thereby understood that the patient was included in the study. Thus, the staff could not be completely blinded to allocation. The researchers performing the baseline interviews could not be blinded. The plan was that the collection of baseline measures and the performance of follow-up interviews were to be carried out by different researchers in order to keep the researchers blinded at the follow-up. However, the participants may have revealed the allocation (i.e., whether administered the CGA or not) during the follow-up interviews, making the interviewers non-blinded. To address this, we added a variable at all follow-ups indicating whether or not the allocation had been revealed which also reflects whether or not the participant was aware of being administered the CGA or not.

Meetings with representatives of all staff categories were regularly held at the intervention ward throughout the entire intervention period. There was a steering group with representatives from the research group and the different clinical care levels (geriatrics, internal medicine and rehabilitation) that met regularly, starting with the planning of the study and lasting throughout the whole study period.

The researchers (occupational therapists, physiotherapists, registered nurses and physicians) performing the interviews and measurements at baseline and follow-ups were all trained in observing and assessing in accordance with the guidelines for the outcome measurements.

2.7. Outcome Measures

For an overview of outcome measures and time of measure, see Table 2.

Table 2. Outcome measures and follow-ups.

Primary Outcomes	Measurement	Baseline	1 Month	6 Months	1 Year
Dependence	ADL-staircase [33]	X	X	X	X
Secondary Outcomes					
Functional status	Timed Up and Go [34]	X	X	X	X
	The Berg Balance Scale [35]	X			X
	Gait Speed 4 m [36]	X	X	X	X
	Grip Strength North Coast Dynamometer [37]	X	X	X	X
Cognition	Mini Mental State Examination (MMSE) [38]	X	X	X	X
Self-rated health	Questionnaire	X	X	X	X
	Symptoms: Göteborg Quality of Life Instrument [39]	X	X	X	X
Life satisfaction	Fugl–Meyer–Lisat-11 Questionnaire [40]	X	X	X	X
Satisfaction with quality of care	Questionnaire	X			
Health care consumption	Register Data				
Home help services	Questionnaire/Register Data	X	X	X	X
Capability	ICECAP-O [41]	X			X
Mortality	Register Data				

2.7.1. The Primary Outcome

Dependence in daily activities was measured using the ADL-staircase assessment [33] by combining both interviews and observations. It includes dependence in nine activities: cleaning, shopping, transportation, cooking, bathing, dressing, going to the toilet, transferring and feeding. Dependence was defined as a state in which another person is involved in the activity by giving personal or directive assistance. The sum of dependence in the nine activities of daily living is calculated, range 0–9, with a clinically significant change of ≥1 unit between baseline and follow-up. At baseline, personal ADL (PADL: bathing, dressing, going to the toilet, transferring and feeding) was inquired for both actual PADL status during the hospital stay and retrospectively for PADL before onset of the acute illness leading to the hospital admission. This was done because the acute illness often leads to a higher dependence in PADL.

2.7.2. The Secondary Outcomes

Functional status was measured using the Timed Up and Go (TUG) test [34], the Berg Balance Scale [35], Gait Speed four-metre walking test [36] and Grip Strength with North Coast Dynamometer [37]. The TUG test measures the time for a person to rise from a chair, walk 3 m, turn around, walk back, and sit down again. It measures both static and dynamic balance. In this study, we defined a change of ≥4 s as a clinically significant difference between baseline and follow-up, with 3.6 s considered as the minimal detectable change for TUG test measurements [42]. For details on Berg Balance Scale, Gait Speed and Grip Strength, see Section 2.8. Cognition was measured using the Mini Mental State Examination [38], see Section 2.8.

Self-rated was measured by the question: "In general, would you say your health is", with the response alternatives: excellent, very good, good, fair, and poor. Clinically significant difference was defined as ≥1 step in the response alternatives between baseline and follow-up. In addition, self-reported symptoms were measured using the Göteborg Quality of Life Instrument [39].

Life satisfaction was measured using the Fugl–Meyer–Lisat-11 Questionnaire [40] which includes 11 items concerning satisfaction with: life as a whole, work, financial situation, leisure, friends and acquaintances, sexual life, functional capacity, family life, partner relationship, physical health and psychological health. Response alternatives included: very dissatisfied, dissatisfied, rather dissatisfied, rather satisfied, satisfied and very satisfied. In the analysis, the responses to each question were dichotomised into satisfied (very satisfied and satisfied) or not satisfied (rather satisfied, rather dissatisfied, dissatisfied and very dissatisfied) as was done in the validation of the questionnaire [40]. The sum of items for which the respondent reported being satisfied were calculated, range 0–11, with a clinically significant change of ≥1 between baseline and follow-up.

Satisfaction with quality of care was measured by the participant's agreement with six statements with a person-centred approach: "I feel that the care given during the hospital stay meets my needs", "I feel that the care planning meeting before discharge was valuable", "I was able to take part in the discussion of my needs in the care planning meeting", "I feel that the actions planned equal my needs", "I feel that the actions delivered equal my needs" and "I am satisfied with the hospital care". The response alternatives were agree completely, agree partly, neither agree nor disagree, disagree, and disagree completely. An answer of agree completely or agree partly were considered as satisfied. These questions were only measured once (at 1 month follow-up) and were used as the difference between intervention and control groups in the proportion of participants being satisfied for each question at follow-up as has been done previously [43].

Outcomes concerning health–economic aspects are health and social care consumption. Data on health care consumption can be retrieved from the regional care databases, including in-hospital and outpatient care, visits to primary healthcare (physicians, physiotherapists, occupational therapists, nurses, and assistant nurses) and home visits by primary healthcare professionals. The number of readmissions, number of in-hospital days, time until first readmission and number of outpatient visits were calculated and compared between intervention and control group for 1 year after study enrolment. Social care consumption was measured by questions about help received for instrumental and personal ADL from the municipality, privately financed help, relatives, friends and/or other. Response alternatives included none, less than once a week, once a week or more and daily. Extent and frequency of help received was calculated and compared between intervention and control groups for 1 year after study enrolment. In addition, questions covered institutional care, such as nursing home, retirement home and sheltered housing, from which the number of days in institutional care were calculated and compared between intervention and control groups for 1 year after study enrolment.

To add to this, we used the ICECAP-O [41,44], which measures capability in older people, for use in the economic evaluation of health and social care interventions. It focuses on well-being defined in a broader sense and covers five attributes: (1) attachment; (2) security; (3) role; (4) enjoyment; and (5) control. The respondent chose one of five statements for each attribute. (1) Attachment: "I can have all the love and friendship that I want"; "I can have a lot of the love and friendship that I want"; "I can have a little of the love and friendship that I want"; "I cannot have any of the love and friendship that I want". (2) Security: "I can think about the future without any concern"; "I can think about the future with only a little concern"; "I can only think about the future with some concern"; "I can only think about the future with a lot of concern". (3) Role: "I am able to do all the things that make me feel valued"; "I am able to do many of the things that make me feel valued"; "I am able to do a few of the things that make me feel valued"; "I am unable to do any of the things that make me feel valued". (4) Enjoyment: "I can have all the enjoyment and pleasure that I want"; "I can have a lot of the enjoyment and pleasure that I want"; "I can have a little of the enjoyment and pleasure that I want"; "I cannot have any of the enjoyment and pleasure that I want". (5) Control: "I am able to be completely independent"; "I am able to be independent in many things"; "I am able to be independent in a few things"; "I am unable to be at all independent".

Mortality rates will be retrieved from the National Cause of Death Registry.

2.8. Measurement of Frailty Indicators

In this study, we used the following measurements and cut-off levels of frailty indicators:

Weakness: Reduced grip strength considered to be below lowest norm range for ages 80–84, 13 kg for women and 21 kg for men for the right hand and below 10 kg for women and 18 kg for men for the left hand, using a North Coast dynamometer [37].

Fatigue: Question from the Göteborg Quality of Life Instrument [39], answering "Yes" to the question "Have you suffered any general fatigue/tiredness over the last three months?"

Weight loss: Question from the Göteborg Quality of Life Instrument [39], answering "Yes" to the question "Have you suffered any weight loss over the last three months?"

Reduced physical activity: Taking 1–2 or less outdoor walks per week.

Impaired balance: The Berg Balance Scale [35,45,46], reduced balance defined as having a value of 47 or less.

Reduced gait speed: Walking four metres with a gait speed of 0.6 metres/second or slower [36].

Visual impairment: The KM chart (Konstantin Moutakis chart) [47], impaired vision defined as having a visual acuity of 0.5 or less.

Impaired cognition: The MMSE [38], impaired cognition defined as having a score below 25.

2.9. Statistical Analysis and Power Calculation

A power calculation was done based on the primary outcome variable, dependence in activities of daily living (range 0–9) with an assumed difference between the intervention and control groups of one dependence (i.e., dependent in one or more activities of daily living, a clinically relevant difference of importance to the individual as well as the caregiver) and a standard deviation of 2 in both groups. To detect a difference between the intervention and control groups with a two-sided test and with a significance level of $\alpha = 0.05$ and 80% power, at least 64 participants were needed in each group. To take a potential loss to follow-up into account, a total of 150 persons (75 in the control group and 75 in the intervention group) were initially planned to be included. This was later revised to allow for a higher loss to follow-up (22%) with 78 + 78, equalling a total of 156 participants. The assumed loss to follow-up and the power calculation were based on previous research on frail older people in need of acute care [48].

Both descriptive and analytical statistics were used in order to compare groups and to analyse changes over time. Non-parametric statistics were used when ordinal data were analysed. Otherwise, parametric statistics were used. Besides descriptive statistics, the chi^2 and Fisher's two-tailed exact tests to test differences in the proportions among the groups were used. A value of $p \leq 0.05$ (two-tailed) were considered significant. The analysis were made on the basis of the intention-to-treat principle, meaning that participants were analysed on the basis of the group to which they were initially randomised. Given the old age of the participants, a relatively high drop-out rate was inevitable. Simply analysing complete cases is not relevant and might lead to bias, especially since missing data would not be at random. Therefore, the approach of data imputation was the replacement of missing values with a value based on the median change of deterioration between baseline and follow-up of all who participated in the follow-up [20]. The reasons for this imputation method were that (1) the study sample (frail older people) was expected to deteriorate over time as a natural course of the ageing process and (2) deteriorated health often is a reason for not fulfilling the follow-ups. Worst-case change was imputed for those who died before follow-up.

2.10. Process Evaluation

The process evaluation aims to provide insight into what is inside "the black box", i.e., shed light on the function and consequences of the intervention—why it works or fails. The process evaluation includes context, recruitment, reach, dose delivered and received and fidelity [49], targeting recruitment and collection of outcome measures during the hospital stay and after discharge. The process evaluation focuses on the following aspects in line with the recommendations of the Medical Research Council [30]:

- The intervention, the actual exposure and the experience of the participants;
- Evaluation of which components of the intervention contributed to its success or failure;
- Description of the conditions under which the intervention is successful/unsuccessful.

The evaluation includes in-depth qualitative interviews with eight to ten participants in the intervention group, focusing on their experiences of receiving care according to the CGA [27]. The experiences of the staff working with to the CGA are explored through focus group discussions in order to gain an understanding of the intervention and its significance as well as its implementation. This includes the respondent's role in working according to the CGA, perceptions about the CGA and its significance and effectiveness and possibilities and challenges involved in working according to the CGA. The focus group methodology distinctly utilises the interaction among participants in order to collect data, encouraging them to clarify not only what they think but also how and why they think in a certain way. The method is suitable for collecting the views and experiences of a selected group and generating a broad knowledge and understanding [50]. In addition, medical records are reviewed to assure that the assessments in the CGA have been conducted as intended, what aspects of CGA has been performed and by whom (i.e., the actual exposure).

2.11. Economic Analysis

The first step in the health–economic evaluation was to conduct a cost-minimisation analysis that compared the total costs between the CGA and CONTROL during the full follow-up period using the healthcare consumption data (measured as the cost of all resources used) as described above. This showed the cost implications for the payers if implementing the CGA or CONTROL.

The second step in the health–economic evaluation was to conduct a cost-effectiveness analysis. The cost-effectiveness of the intervention (versus the control) was evaluated based on the incremental cost-effectiveness ratio (ICER): ICER = (CostCGA − CostCONTROL)/(EffectivenessCGA − EffectivenessCONTROL). The effectiveness measure was based on the score from the ICECAP-O which measures older people's capability for use in economic evaluation [41,44]. The ICER can be interpreted as the cost per one-unit gain in full capability and can, as such, be compared to other interventions using the same outcome measure in order to evaluate the relative cost-effectiveness. Sensitivity analysis and confidence intervals were calculated based on the non-parametric bootstrap approach.

2.12. Time Plan of the Study

The inclusion began in March 2016 and was completed in December 2018. The intervention began when the participant was admitted to the ward and lasted until discharge from the hospital. The follow-ups after one year are planned to be completed in January 2020. See Table 3 for time plan for the study and follow-ups.

Table 3. Time plan for the study and follow-ups.

	Started	Completed	To Be Completed
Inclusion	March 2016	December 2018	
Baseline	March 2016	December 2018	
1 month follow-up	April 2016	January 2019	
6 month follow-up	September 2016	July 2019	
12 month follow-up	March 2016		January 2020

3. Results

3.1. Baseline Characteristics

The inclusion and randomisation were carried out by the hospital bed coordinators at the emergency departments, because they are always involved when a patient is admitted to a ward, and they are responsible for coordinating available hospital beds. They had no extra time for this task and presumably did not always remember to inform and ask eligible patients. In addition, in many cases it was not possible to randomise due to the shortage of hospital beds at the wards (as there had to be a vacant bed at both the intervention ward and the control ward to be able to randomise). We asked the hospital bed coordinators to monitor how many patients were eligible and how many declined to participate. Unfortunately, due to their high work load, they only monitored this for approximately half a year. Based on the monitoring that was conducted, we estimated that approximately 210 eligible patients were asked to participate, and 178 of those consented to participate resulting in an estimated participation rate of approximately 85%. For details regarding the number of participants receiving allocated intervention with baseline data and reasons for declining participation, see Figure 2.

The median age of the participants in the inclusion year was 87 years in the control and 87.5 years in the intervention group. There were no statistically significant differences concerning baseline characteristics, frailty indicators and ADL between the control and intervention groups, see Tables 4–6.

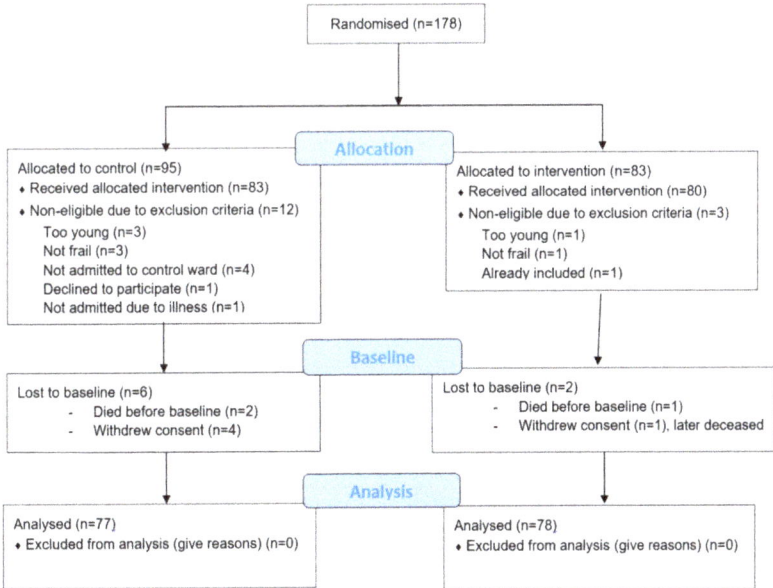

Figure 2. Flowchart of the three phases of the study implementing the "Comprehensive Geriatric Assessment in Swedish Acute Hospital Settings (CGA-Swed): A Randomised Controlled Study", according to CONSORT [28].

Table 4. Baseline characteristics of the study population.

Characteristics	Control Group N = 77	Intervention Group N = 78	p-Value
Age, mean (range)	86.2 (76–98)	87.5 (75–101)	0.17
Female, % (n)	55.8 (43)	60.3 (47)	0.58
Living alone, % (n)	62.3 (48)	65.4 (51)	0.70
Academic education, % (n)	20.1 (16)	10.3 (8)	0.07
Good self-rated health, % (n) *	27.3 (21)	33.3 (26)	0.41
CIRS-G ≥ 3 in any category, % **	93.5 (72)	98.7 (77)	0.26
CIRS-G, median number of ratings 3–4 (range)	3 (0–9)	3 (0–7)	

* Excellent, very good or good. ** Cumulative Illness Rating Scale for Geriatrics. Rating 3 = severe/constant significant disability/uncontrollable chronic problem and rating 4 = extremely severe/immediate treatment required/end-organ failure/severe impairment in function [51].

Table 5. Frailty indicators.

Frailty Indicator	Control Group N = 77	Intervention group N = 78	p-Value
Fatigue, % (n) [1]	90.9 (70)	87.2 (68)	0.46
Weight loss, % (n) [2]	50.0 (38)	51.9 (40)	0.81
Weakness, % (n) [3]	28.6 (22)	36.0 (27)	0.33
Reduced physical activity, % (n) [4]	71.1 (54)	68.0 (51)	0.68
Impaired balance, % (n) [5]	86.8 (66)	94.8 (73)	0.09
Reduced gait speed, % (n) [6]	75.3 (58)	84.2 (64)	0.17
Visual impairment, % (n) [7]	80.0 (60)	78.7 (59)	0.84
Impaired cognition, % (n) [8]	48.1 (37)	52.0 (39)	0.63
Number of frailty indicators [9]			
1, % (n)	1.3 (1)	0	0.88
2, % (n)	6.5 (5)	3.8 (3)	
3, % (n)	11.7 (9)	9.0 (7)	
4, % (n)	11.7 (9)	14.1 (11)	
5, % (n)	19.5 (15)	21.8 (17)	
6, % (n)	20.8 (16)	26.9 (21)	
7, % (n)	20.8 (16)	16.7 (13)	
8, % (n)	7.8 (6)	7.7 (6)	

[1] Answering "Yes" to the question "Have you suffered any general fatigue/tiredness over the last three months?" (Part of the Göteborg Quality of Life Instrument [39]). [2] Answering "Yes" to the question "Have you suffered any weight loss over the last three months?" (Part of the Göteborg Quality of Life Instrument [39]). Missing 1 in the control. [3] Reduced grip strength: below 13 kg for women and 21 kg for men for the right hand and below 10 kg for women and 18 kg for men for the left hand, using a North Coast dynamometer [37]. Missing 3 in the intervention. [4] Taking outdoor walks 1–2 times a week or less. Missing 1 in the control and 3 in the intervention. [5] Having a value of 47 or less on the Berg Balance Scale [35,45,46]. Missing 1 in the control and 1 in the intervention. [6] Walking four metres with a gait speed of 0.6 metres/second or slower [36]. Missing 2 in the control and 2 in the intervention. [7] Having a visual acuity of 0.5 or less using the KM chart [47]. Missing 2 in the control and 3 in the intervention. [8] Scoring below 25 on the Mini Mental State Examination (MMSE) [38]. Missing 3 in the intervention. [9] Missing information on 1–4 frailty indicators for 13 participants.

3.2. Process Evaluation during Inclusion Period

There was a period (approximately half a year) with very high work strain for the CGA staff during the inclusion. The ward had to open up ten additional hospital beds within a couple of days due to the shortage of beds available at the hospital. This led to the need of hiring staff that did not have the knowledge and experience of working according to the CGA. Therefore, it is probable that a majority of the participants in the intervention group during this period did not receive a full CGA. Through the medical record review, we will investigate the extent to which the CGA was documented for each participant in order to be able to estimate the completeness of the CGA actually received by each participant in the intervention group.

In addition, there have been many readmissions during the follow-up period, in many cases to a different ward than during the inclusion. Thus, several participants in the control group may have received care at the CGA ward during the year after inclusion. This also needs to be considered when analysing follow-up data.

Table 6. ADL dependence at baseline.

Number of Dependences		Control Group N = 77	Intervention Group N = 78	p-Value
IADL dependence, % (n)	0	9.1 (7)	6.4 (5)	0.11
	1	19.5 (15)	7.7 (6)	
	2	18.2 (14)	14.1 (11)	
	3	20.8 (16)	21.8 (17)	
	4	32.5 (25)	50.0 (39)	
PADL dependence before onset of illness, % (n)	0	61.0 (47)	52.6 (41)	0.83
	1	15.6 (12)	16.7 (13)	
	2	7.8 (6)	12.8 (10)	
	3	7.8 (6)	7.7 (6)	
	4	5.2 (4)	5.1 (4)	
	5	2.6 (2)	5.1 (4)	
PADL dependence during hospital stay, % (n)	0	31.2 (24)	23.1 (18)	0.38
	1	20.8 (16)	11.5 (9)	
	2	9.1 (7)	12.8 (10)	
	3	9.1 (7)	10.3 (8)	
	4	24.7 (19)	33.3 (26)	
	5	5.2 (4)	9.0 (7)	

4. Discussion

The study "CGA-Swed" was designed to evaluate the effects of the CGA for frail older people in Swedish acute hospital settings. The primary outcome was dependence in ADL, as this has been pointed out as an important aspect for frail older people in previous research [52,53]. Secondary outcomes include other important aspects and patient-related outcomes such as self-rated health, life satisfaction, satisfaction with care, health care consumption and cost-effectiveness. Another strength of the study was the process evaluation alongside the RCT, adding to the knowledge on the implementation of the CGA and, thus, filling a knowledge gap pointed out by the Cochrane reviews of the CGA [9,10].

The randomisation seems to have been successful, as the baseline characteristics were similar between the intervention and control groups with no statistically significant differences among the two groups. Unfortunately, we do not know how many eligible participants could have been asked to participate nor how many in fact were asked to participate. This limitation could be seen as a consequence of performing a complex intervention in "real life", being dependent on clinical staff performing parts of the research process. In our study, we were dependent on the hospital bed coordinators asking eligible participants beyond their ordinary duties as hospital bed coordinators and with no extra time or reward given. Similarly, it was not possible for us to have a researcher designated for the inclusion, since this would have required too much time and resources. Our estimate of a participation rate of 85% may seem high but seems realistic to us after discussion with the hospital bed coordinators. However, some of the participants had not fully understood what they had consented to, as they were asked about participation when seeking care for an acute medical problem. There is a risk that some were so comforted by being admitted to a ward that they consented out of pure relief. However, the researcher doing the baseline interview repeated the information about the study and asked once again about consent to participate, and very few participants declined participation at this occasion.

The baseline characteristics show that our sample was frail and had a high morbidity and high degree of dependence in activities of daily living. This is not surprising, since they all were screened as frail and in need of acute in-hospital care. The prevalence of frailty is known to be high among patients in internal medicine wards and especially in geriatric wards [54]. Thus, we argue that our sample is representative for frail older hospital medical in-patients. However, this also indicates a risk of high mortality within the sample, as both frailty and comorbidity are risk factors for high mortality [3,55]. Already during the hospital stay, three participants died, and preliminary data shows a high mortality rate to the follow-ups, higher than we expected based on earlier research [22,48].

The implementation process evaluation alongside the RCT—aiming to provide insight into the function and consequences of the intervention, why it works or fails—is an important part of the design that will contribute with insights into real-life conditions that may be challenging in implementing the CGA. The logistics of the intervention and the research procedures were tested in the pilot study and were found feasible [26]. The major deviation from the plan was the prolonged inclusion period because of the lack of available hospital beds which has prevailed throughout the study. However, we were eventually able to include the first estimated sample size of 150 participants, lacking only one participant to reach the revised estimated sample size of 156 participants. The process evaluation is a strength of the study, enabling us to generate knowledge on the process of the implementation of the CGA which has been pointed out as a knowledge gap by the Cochrane reviews of the CGA [9,10]. The results of the implementation process evaluation are planned to be presented in a forthcoming paper. There were some obvious threats to the study during the inclusion period and the follow-up period that we already observed and which may hamper our ability to demonstrate positive outcomes. The period with high work strain at the intervention ward is very likely to have led to CGAs of both lower quantity and quality than what was planned for. The patient medical record review will help us identify those not receiving a full CGA and allow us to adjust the analysis accordingly. However, this will probably lead to lower ability to detect a true difference between the groups. In addition, the fact that participants in the control group might have been admitted to the intervention group during the follow-up period needs to be accounted for in the analysis. As this can make the sample in each group smaller, this might also lead to lower power.

Findings on how frail older persons experience receiving care according to the CGA have already been published elsewhere based on this study, showing that they experienced being seen as a person while being admitted to a CGA ward [27].

To a large extent, we used the same questionnaires, measurements, manuals and outcomes as in our previous studies "Elderly Persons in the Risk Zone" [56] and "Continuum of Care for Frail Elderly People" [48]. This gives us the opportunity to compare among the studies with different levels of frailty within the samples, with the sample in "Elderly Persons in the Risk Zone" being prefrail [56] and the sample in "Continuum of Care" being less frail [48] than the sample in the current study. The outcome measures for the studies were carefully selected to make sure that they are valid and reliable for the target group and covering different components and levels of frailty.

We planned to have different researchers doing the baseline interviews and the follow-ups so as to be able to keep the researcher blinded at the follow-ups. However, in many cases it has been and will be the same research assistant doing the follow-up interviews who also conducted the baseline interview. Thus, we have not been able to keep the researcher blinded at the follow-up. The research assistant has, however, conducted most of the baseline interviews ($n = 155$) and in most cases did not remember the group assignment. It can also be seen as a strength that the same person carries out most interviews and assessments, as this ensures that the questions and assessments are done similarly at all occasions, thus enhancing the reliability of the assessments. In addition, having the same person in the follow-ups minimises the number of persons the participant has to meet. This might increase the chance of the participant remaining in the study, as they already are familiar with the person asking to do the follow-up. Since we had a variable at the follow-up regarding whether or not the researcher was aware of the allocation or whether the participant had revealed the allocation during the interview, we will know to what extent the researcher was blinded.

The intervention was planned in collaboration with representatives from the Department of Geriatrics (i.e., intervention ward), the Department of Medicine (i.e., control wards) and the Department of Occupational Therapy and Physiotherapy. Regular meetings were held, starting with the planning of the study and lasting throughout the intervention period to discuss the content of the intervention and the research procedures which enhanced the implementation and strengthened the study. Both the research group and the group of professionals carrying out the intervention are multi-professional which is important since the CGA implies multi-professional team collaboration.

In summary, this study evaluated the CGA in current Swedish acute hospital settings employing a randomised controlled design, adding to the knowledge of the effects of the CGA in today's hospital care which is characterised by shorter hospital stays and fewer available hospital beds than before. The results are expected to optimise the implementation of future complex interventions and lead to the improvement of care, support and rehabilitation of frail older people with complex needs. The process evaluation, aiming to provide insights into the function and consequences of the intervention—why it works or fails—is an important part of the design that will contribute with insights into real life conditions that may be challenging in implementing the CGA. This study is expected to show positive effects on frail older people's dependence in activities of daily living, an outcome that is important for both the person and society. In addition, the CGA has potential to increase the satisfaction with care, life satisfaction and self-rated health as well as prevent deterioration in functional status and to be cost effective.

Author Contributions: K.W. led the intervention of the study and was the primary author of the manuscript. K.W., A.E. and S.D.I. participated in the research design. K.W., A.E., J.N., J.E., N.E. and S.D.I. participated in the planning of the study. K.W., I.A.H., T.W., E.H., N.D.Å. and S.D.I. participated in the implementation of the study. K.W., I.A.H., T.W. and E.H. collected data. All authors contributed to the writing and review of the manuscript and approved the submitted version of the manuscript. All authors have read and agreed to the published version of the manuscript.

Funding: This study was funded by grants from FORTE (registration number 2015-00043), the Swedish state under the agreement between the Swedish government and the county councils (the ALF-agreement, ALFBGB-530971/-673831/-716571) and Region Västra Götaland, Department of Research and Development (VGFOUREG-565511/-63881/-736281) and The King Gustav and Queen Victoria Freemasons Foundation.

Acknowledgments: Special thanks to the hospital bed coordinators at Sahlgrenska University Hospital, Catarina Söderström and Jenny Midsem, for their participation in the inclusion of participants, and to research assistant Katharina Sjöberg for data collection.

Conflicts of Interest: The authors declare no conflict of interest.

References

1. Barber, R.M.; Fullman, N.; Sorensen, R.J.; Bollyky, T.; McKee, M.; Nolte, E.; Abajobir, A.A.; Abate, K.H.; Abbafati, C.; Abbas, K.M. Healthcare Access and Quality Index based on mortality from causes amenable to personal health care in 195 countries and territories, 1990–2015: A novel analysis from the Global Burden of Disease Study 2015. *Lancet* **2017**, *390*, 231–266. [CrossRef]
2. Lafont, C.; Gérard, S.; Voisin, T.; Pahor, M.; Vellas, B. Reducing "iatrogenic disability" in the hospitalized frail elderly. *J. Nutr. Health Aging* **2011**, *15*, 645–660. [CrossRef] [PubMed]
3. Morley, J.E.; Vellas, B.; Van Kan, G.A.; Anker, S.D.; Bauer, J.M.; Bernabei, R.; Cesari, M.; Chumlea, W.; Doehner, W.; Evans, J. Frailty consensus: A call to action. *J. Am. Med. Dir. Assoc.* **2013**, *14*, 392–397. [CrossRef] [PubMed]
4. McMillan, G.; Hubbard, R. Frailty in older inpatients: What physicians need to know. *QJM Int. J. Med.* **2012**, *105*, 1059–1065. [CrossRef] [PubMed]
5. Clegg, A.; Young, J.; Iliffe, S.; Rikkert, M.O.; Rockwood, K. Frailty in elderly people. *Lancet* **2013**, *381*, 752–762. [CrossRef]
6. Castell, M.V.; Van Der Pas, S.; Otero, A.; Siviero, P.; Dennison, E.; Denkinger, M.; Pedersen, N.; Sanchez-Martinez, M.; Queipo, R.; Van Schoor, N. Osteoarthritis and frailty in elderly individuals across six European countries: Results from the European Project on OSteoArthritis (EPOSA). *BMC Musculoskelet. Dis.* **2015**, *16*, 359. [CrossRef] [PubMed]
7. Haider, S.; Grabovac, I.; Dorner, T.E. Fulfillment of physical activity guidelines in the general population and frailty status in the elderly population. *Wiener Klin. Wochenschr.* **2019**, *131*, 288–293. [CrossRef]

8. Ekdahl, A.; Sjöstrand, F.; Ehrenberg, A.; Oredsson, S.; Stavenow, L.; Wisten, A.; Wårdh, I.; Ivanoff, S.D. Frailty and comprehensive geriatric assessment organized as CGA-ward or CGA-consult for older adult patients in the acute care setting: A systematic review and meta-analysis. *Eur. Geriatr. Med.* **2015**, *6*, 523–540. [CrossRef]
9. Ellis, G.; Gardner, M.; Tsiachristas, A.; Langhorne, P.; Burke, O.; Harwood, R.H.; Conroy, S.P.; Kircher, T.; Somme, D.; Saltvedt, I. Comprehensive geriatric assessment for older adults admitted to hospital. *Cochrane Database Syst. Rev.* **2017**. [CrossRef]
10. Ellis, G.; Whitehead, M.A.; Robinson, D.; O'Neill, D.; Langhorne, P. Comprehensive geriatric assessment for older adults admitted to hospital: Meta-analysis of randomised controlled trials. *BMJ* **2011**, *343*, d6553. [CrossRef]
11. Swedish Agency for Health Technology Assessment and Assessment of Social Services. Comprehensive Geriatric Assessment and Care of Frail Elderly. SBU Report no 221. 2014. Available online: https://www.sbu.se/sv/publikationer/SBU-utvarderar/omhandertagande-av-aldre-som-inkommer-akut-till-sjukhus--med-fokus-pa-skora-aldre/ (accessed on 9 December 2019). (In Swedish)
12. Barnes, D.E.; Palmer, R.M.; Kresevic, D.M.; Fortinsky, R.H.; Kowal, J.; Chren, M.-M.; Landefeld, C.S. Acute care for elders units produced shorter hospital stays at lower cost while maintaining patients' functional status. *Health Aff.* **2012**, *31*, 1227–1236. [CrossRef] [PubMed]
13. Ekerstad, N.; Karlson, B.W.; Andersson, D.; Husberg, M.; Carlsson, P.; Heintz, E.; Alwin, J. Short-term resource utilization and cost-effectiveness of comprehensive geriatric assessment in acute hospital care for severely frail elderly patients. *J. Am. Med. Dir. Assoc.* **2018**, *19*, 871–878.e872. [CrossRef] [PubMed]
14. Melis, R.J.; Adang, E.; Teerenstra, S.; van Eijken, M.I.; Wimo, A.; Achterberg, T.V.; Lisdonk, E.H.V.d.; Rikkert, M.G.O. Multidimensional geriatric assessment: Back to the future cost-effectiveness of a multi-disciplinary intervention model for community-dwelling frail older people. *J. Gerontol A Biol. Sci. Med. Sci* **2008**, *63*, 275–282. [CrossRef] [PubMed]
15. Rubenstein, L.; Siu, A.; Wieland, D. Comprehensive geriatric assessment: Toward understanding its efficacy. *Aging Clin. Exp. Res.* **1989**, *1*, 87–98. [CrossRef]
16. Gladman, J.R.; Conroy, S.P.; Ranhoff, A.H.; Gordon, A.L. New horizons in the implementation and research of comprehensive geriatric assessment: Knowing, doing and the 'know-do'gap. *Age Ageing* **2016**, *45*, 194–200. [CrossRef]
17. Graf, C.E.; Zekry, D.; Giannelli, S.; Michel, J.-P.; Chevalley, T. Efficiency and applicability of comprehensive geriatric assessment in the emergency department: A systematic review. *Aging Clin. Exp. Res.* **2011**, *23*, 244–254. [CrossRef]
18. Leichsenring, K. Developing integrated health and social care services for older persons in Europe. *Int. J. Integr. Care* **2004**, *4*. [CrossRef]
19. Eklund, K.; Wilhelmson, K.; Landahl, S.; Ivanoff-Dahlin, S. Screening for frailty among older emergency department visitors: Validation of the new FRESH-screening instrument. *BMC Emerg. Med.* **2016**, *16*, 27. [CrossRef]
20. OECD. Health Statistics. Available online: http://www.oecd.org/els/health-systems/health-data.htm (accessed on 30 August 2017).
21. Borgström, A. Sverige har lägst antalet vårdplatser i Europa. [Sweden has the lowest number of hospital beds in Europe]. *Läkartidningen* **2007**, *104*, 396–397.
22. Eklund, K.; Wilhelmson, K.; Gustafsson, H.; Landahl, S.; Dahlin-Ivanoff, S. One-year outcome of frailty indicators and activities of daily living following the randomised controlled trial: "Continuum of care for frail older people". *BMC Geriatr.* **2013**, *13*, 76. [CrossRef]
23. Ekdahl, A.W.; Alwin, J.; Eckerblad, J.; Husberg, M.; Jaarsma, T.; Mazya, A.L.; Milberg, A.; Krevers, B.; Unosson, M.; Wiklund, R. Long-term evaluation of the ambulatory geriatric assessment: A frailty intervention trial (AGe-FIT): Clinical outcomes and total costs after 36 months. *J. Am. Med. Dir. Assoc.* **2016**, *17*, 263–268. [CrossRef] [PubMed]
24. Ekerstad, N.; Karlson, B.W.; Ivanoff, S.D.; Landahl, S.; Andersson, D.; Heintz, E.; Husberg, M.; Alwin, J. Is the acute care of frail elderly patients in a comprehensive geriatric assessment unit superior to conventional acute medical care? *Clin. Interv. Aging* **2017**, *12*, 1. [CrossRef] [PubMed]
25. Parker, S.; McCue, P.; Phelps, K.; McCleod, A.; Arora, S.; Nockels, K.; Kennedy, S.; Roberts, H.; Conroy, S. What is comprehensive geriatric assessment (CGA)? An umbrella review. *Age Ageing* **2017**, *47*, 149–155. [CrossRef] [PubMed]

26. Westgård, T.; Ottenvall Hammar, I.; Holmgren, E.; Ehrenberg, A.; Wisten, A.; Ekdahl, A.W.; Dahlin-Ivanoff, S.; Wilhelmson, K. Comprehensive geriatric assessment pilot of a randomized control study in a Swedish acute hospital: A feasibility study. *Pilot Feasibility Stud.* **2018**, *4*, 41. [CrossRef]
27. Westgård, T.; Wilhelmson, K.; Dahlin-Ivanoff, S.; Ottenvall Hammar, I. Feeling Respected as a Person: A Qualitative Analysis of Frail Older People's Experiences on an Acute Geriatric Ward Practicing a Comprehensive Geriatric Assessment. *Geriatrics* **2019**, *4*, 16. [CrossRef]
28. Zwarenstein, M.; Treweek, S.; Gagnier, J.J.; Altman, D.G.; Tunis, S.; Haynes, B.; Oxman, A.D.; Moher, D. Improving the reporting of pragmatic trials: An extension of the CONSORT statement. *BMJ* **2008**, *337*, a2390. [CrossRef]
29. Statistics Sweden. Available online: http://www.statistikdatabasen.scb.se (accessed on 28 October 2019).
30. Medical Resarch Council. Available online: http://www.mrc.ac.uk/ (accessed on 30 August 2017).
31. Ekman, I.; Swedberg, K.; Taft, C.; Lindseth, A.; Norberg, A.; Brink, E.; Carlsson, J.; Dahlin-Ivanoff, S.; Johansson, I.-L.; Kjellgren, K. Person-centered care—Ready for prime time. *Eur. J. Cardiovasc. Nurs.* **2011**, *10*, 248–251. [CrossRef]
32. GraphPad. Random Number Generator. Available online: https://graphpad.com/quickcalcs/randomN1.cfm (accessed on 9 December 2019).
33. Sonn, U. Longitudinal studies of dependence in daily life activities among elderly persons. *Scand. J. Rehabil. Med. Suppl.* **1996**, *34*, 1–35.
34. Schoppen, T.; Boonstra, A.; Groothoff, J.W.; de Vries, J.; Göeken, L.N.; Eisma, W.H. The Timed "up and go" test: Reliability and validity in persons with unilateral lower limb amputation. *Arch. Phys. Med. Rehabil.* **1999**, *80*, 825–828. [CrossRef]
35. Berg, K.O.; Wood-Dauphinee, S.L.; Williams, J.I.; Maki, B. Measuring balance in the elderly: Validation of an instrument. *Can. J. Public Health* **1992**, *83*, S7–S11. [PubMed]
36. Peterson, M.J.; Giuliani, C.; Morey, M.C.; Pieper, C.F.; Evenson, K.R.; Mercer, V.; Cohen, H.J.; Visser, M.; Brach, J.S.; Kritchevsky, S.B. Physical activity as a preventative factor for frailty: The health, aging, and body composition study. *J. Gerontol. A Biol. Sci. Med. Sci.* **2009**, *64*, 61–68. [CrossRef] [PubMed]
37. Mathiowetz, V.; Kashman, N.; Volland, G.; Weber, K.; Dowe, M.; Rogers, S. Grip and pinch strength: Normative data for adults. *Arch. Phys. Med. Rehabil.* **1985**, *66*, 69–74.
38. Folstein, M.F.; Folstein, S.E.; McHugh, P.R. "Mini-mental state". A practical method for grading the cognitive state of patients for the clinician. *J. Psychiatr. Res.* **1975**, *12*, 189–198. [CrossRef]
39. Tibblin, G.; Tibblin, B.; Peciva, S.; Kullman, S.; Svardsudd, K. "The Goteborg quality of life instrument"–an assessment of well-being and symptoms among men born 1913 and 1923. Methods and validity. *Scand. J. Prim. Health Care. Suppl.* **1990**, *1*, 33–38.
40. Fugl-Meyer, A.R.; Bränholm, I.-B.; Fugl-Meyer, K.S. Happiness and domain-specific life satisfaction in adult northern Swedes. *Clin. Rehabil.* **1991**, *5*, 25–33. [CrossRef]
41. Coast, J.; Peters, T.J.; Natarajan, L.; Sproston, K.; Flynn, T. An assessment of the construct validity of the descriptive system for the ICECAP capability measure for older people. *Qual Life Res.* **2008**, *17*, 967–976. [CrossRef]
42. Resnik, L.; Borgia, M. Reliability of outcome measures for people with lower-limb amputations: Distinguishing true change from statistical error. *Phys. Ther.* **2011**, *91*, 555–565. [CrossRef]
43. Berglund, H.; Wilhelmson, K.; Blomberg, S.; Duner, A.; Kjellgren, K.; Hasson, H. Older people's views of quality of care: A randomised controlled study of continuum of care. *J. Clin. Nurs.* **2013**, *22*, 2934–2944. [CrossRef]
44. Gustafsson, S.; Hörder, H.; Hammar, I.O.; Skoog, I. Face and content validity and acceptability of the Swedish ICECAP-O capability measure: Cognitive interviews with 70-year-old persons. *Health Psychol. Res.* **2018**, *6*, 6496. [CrossRef]
45. Berg, K.; Wood-Dauphine, S.; Williams, J.; Gayton, D. Measuring balance in the elderly: Preliminary development of an instrument. *Physiother. Can.* **1989**, *41*, 304–311. [CrossRef]
46. Chiu, A.Y.; Au-Yeung, S.S.; Lo, S.K. A comparison of four functional tests in discriminating fallers from non-fallers in older people. *Disabil. Rehabil.* **2003**, *25*, 45–50. [CrossRef]
47. Moutakis, K.; Stigmar, G.; Hall-Lindberg, J. Using the KM visual acuity chart for more reliable evaluation of amblyopia compared to the HVOT method. *Acta Ophthalmol. Scand.* **2004**, *82*, 547–551. [CrossRef]

48. Wilhelmson, K.; Duner, A.; Eklund, K.; Gosman-Hedström, G.; Blomberg, S.; Hasson, H.; Gustafsson, H.; Landahl, S.; Dahlin-Ivanoff, S. Design of a randomized controlled study of a multi-professional and multidimensional intervention targeting frail elderly people. *BMC Geriatr.* **2011**, *11*, 24. [CrossRef] [PubMed]
49. Linnan, L.; Steckler, A. *Process. Evaluation for Public Health Interventions and Research*; Jossey-Bass: San Francisco, CA, USA, 2002.
50. Kitzinger, J. The methodology of focus groups: The importance of interaction between research participants. *Sociol. Health Illn.* **1994**, *16*, 103–121. [CrossRef]
51. Miller, M.D.; Paradis, C.F.; Houck, P.R.; Mazumdar, S.; Stack, J.A.; Rifai, A.H.; Mulsant, B.; Reynolds, C.F., 3rd. Rating chronic medical illness burden in geropsychiatric practice and research: Application of the Cumulative Illness Rating Scale. *Psychiatry Res.* **1992**, *41*, 237–248. [CrossRef]
52. Haak, M.; Fange, A.; Iwarsson, S.; Ivanoff, S.D. Home as a signification of independence and autonomy: Experiences among very old Swedish people. *Scand. J. Occup. Ther.* **2007**, *14*, 16–24. [CrossRef]
53. Häggblom-Kronlöf, G.; Hultberg, J.; Eriksson, B.G.; Sonn, U. Experiences of daily occupations at 99 years of age. *Scand. J. Occup. Ther.* **2007**, *14*, 192–200. [CrossRef]
54. Andela, R.M.; Dijkstra, A.; Slaets, J.P.; Sanderman, R. Prevalence of frailty on clinical wards: Description and implications. *Int. J. Nurs. Pract.* **2010**, *16*, 14–19. [CrossRef]
55. Nunes, B.P.; Flores, T.R.; Mielke, G.I.; Thume, E.; Facchini, L.A. Multimorbidity and mortality in older adults: A systematic review and meta-analysis. *Arch. Gerontol. Geriatr.* **2016**, *67*, 130–138. [CrossRef]
56. Dahlin-Ivanoff, S.; Gosman-Hedstrom, G.; Edberg, A.K.; Wilhelmson, K.; Eklund, K.; Duner, A.; Ziden, L.; Welmer, A.K.; Landahl, S. Elderly persons in the risk zone. Design of a multidimensional, health-promoting, randomised three-armed controlled trial for "prefrail" people of 80+ years living at home. *BMC Geriatr.* **2010**, *10*, 27. [CrossRef] [PubMed]

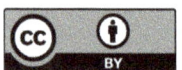

© 2020 by the authors. Licensee MDPI, Basel, Switzerland. This article is an open access article distributed under the terms and conditions of the Creative Commons Attribution (CC BY) license (http://creativecommons.org/licenses/by/4.0/).

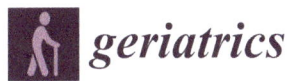

Article

Feeling Respected as a Person: a Qualitative Analysis of Frail Older People's Experiences on an Acute Geriatric Ward Practicing a Comprehensive Geriatric Assessment

Theresa Westgård [1,2,*], Katarina Wilhelmson [1,2,3], Synneve Dahlin-Ivanoff [1,2] and Isabelle Ottenvall Hammar [1,2,4]

1. Department of Health and Rehabilitation, Institute of Neuroscience and Physiology, The Sahlgrenska Academy, University of Gothenburg, 40530 Gothenburg, Sweden; Katarina.wilhelmson@gu.se (K.W.); Synneve.dahlin-ivanoff@neuro.gu.se (S.D.-I.); isabelle.o-h@neuro.gu.se (I.O.H.)
2. Centre of Aging and Health-AGECAP, University of Gothenburg, 40530 Gothenburg, Sweden
3. Department of Geriatrics, The Sahlgrenska University Hospital, 40530 Gothenburg, Sweden
4. Department of Occupational Therapy and Physiotherapy, The Sahlgrenska University Hospital, 40530 Gothenburg, Sweden
* Correspondence: Theresa.westgard@neuro.gu.se

Received: 18 December 2018; Accepted: 24 January 2019; Published: 25 January 2019

Abstract: Comprehensive geriatric assessment (CGA) practices multidimensional, interdisciplinary, and diagnostic processes as a means to identify care needs, plan care, and improve outcomes of frail older people. Conventional content analysis was used to analyze frail older people's experiences of receiving CGA. Through a secondary analysis, interviews and transcripts were revisited in an attempt to discover the meaning behind the participants' implied, ambiguous, and verbalized thoughts that were not illuminated in the primary study. Feeling "respected as a person" is the phenomenon participants described on a CGA acute geriatric ward, achieved by having a reciprocal relationship with the ward staff, enabling their participation in decisions when engaged in communication and understanding. However, when a person was too ill to participate, then care was person-supportive care. CGA, when delivered by staff practicing person-centered care, can keep the frail older person in focus despite them being a patient. If a person-centered care approach does not work because the person is too ill, then person-supportive care is delivered. However, when staff and/or organizational practices do not implement a person-centered care approach, this can hinder patients feeling "respected as a person".

Keywords: geriatric; frail older people; person-centered care; participation; communication; understanding

1. Introduction

Health care services are a fundamental right for all Swedish citizens [1], yet many frail older people requiring acute medical care are faced with a poorly adapted organization of services [2]. These services do not meet the needs of frail older people who present with decreased function, multi-morbidity, and chronic diseases [3–5]. Frailty is related to a deterioration of multiple physiological systems in old age [6]. Symptoms can range from mild to severe, may be dynamic [7], and may have a major impact on quality of life and disability [8] as they are typically associated with restricted activity and morbidity [7]. The literature remains inconsistent with an exact definition of frailty; however, a practiced consensus used in this study follows the operational criteria that: mobility, muscle strength, balance, motor processing, cognition, nutrition, endurance, and physical activity [3] are affected.

Treating frail older people—A complex patient group—Is a challenge for healthcare delivery [9]. When services lack geriatric competence and are not adapted to address the frail older person requiring hospital admission, there is a risk of being marginalized [10].

Therefore frail older people require a comprehensive geriatric assessment (CGA) [11], which is person-centered in praxis if they are to achieve active aging [12] allowing for their well-being. In order to improve the care of frail older people it is important to consider how they experience receiving CGA. CGA is the coordination of a multidisciplinary team that provides multi-dimensional diagnostic and therapeutic processes which are conducted to determine the medical, mental, and functional problems of frail older people so that a coordinated and integrated plan for treatment and follow-up can be developed. By encompassing the whole person, physiological, psychological, and social aspects related to an individual's cumulative disease status and disability are addressed. Results of implementing a CGA model have found that older patients who received the assessment in hospital had increased safety measures documented compared with acute medical wards [13] and were more likely to be alive and in their own homes at follow-up [14]. When examining the CGA team members practicing in a hospital setting, it was identified that quality geriatric care was essentially linked to the assessment process, as this proved to be an interactive, proactive, and a non-hierarchical holistic care approach [15]. CGA is designed to enable frail older people an opportunity to feel safe, trust, and involvement in decision-making while actively aging as recommended by the World Health Organization's (WHO) framework that is based on the principles of health, participation, and security [12].

CGA is designed to include practicing person-centeredness, an approach first coined by Carl Rogers [16], which places the person at the center of their own care. People are granted a position or role that is established by another person/group of persons who ensure a facilitating environment. Once in this environment, the person receives support and is enabled so they can draw strength from their own capabilities while contributing to their care through shared decision-making, equality, and mutual respect [16–18]. Person-centered care involves acknowledging, valuing, and trusting, and is an approach which is considered humanistic, dignified, and morally ethical [17,18]. Person-centered care entails getting to know the unique person, allocation of power and accountability, approachability, and flexibility by organizing and integrating the care directed towards a person's unique values base [19].

Qualitative research on patient's experiences of receiving CGA is sparse. One of the few studies exploring frail older people's experiences of a CGA focused on their illness and limitations related to aging [20]. Another found that inpatient CGA recipients thought that they were merely being monitored and observed, rather than being actively treated while in the hospital, and highlighted that unresolved activities of daily living (ADL) and health needs remained despite being discharged after having received intervention from a geriatrician [21]. As far as we know, the experiences of the frail older people who received a CGA on an acute geriatric medical ward have not been studied in order to understand the underlying meaning of how they experienced their care. Therefore, the aim of this study is to explore how frail older people experienced receiving CGA on an acute geriatric medical ward.

2. Methods

Conventional content analysis is largely used with a study design whose aim is to discover the phenomenon [22], as in the case of this study where research is sparse, limited, and undeveloped. In the present study, a secondary analysis of qualitative data previously used for a narrative analysis was used. The primary data analysis explored how occupations and experiences of frail older people influenced their understanding of health and medical care services (forthcoming paper). The present study revisits the interviews and transcripts of the frail older people to explore how they experienced receiving CGA on an acute geriatric ward. Conventional content analysis is a method designed to objectify the process of inferences, which are deeper than the literal surface level related to the data initially uncovered about the people, social processes, and the situations experienced [23].

2.1. Setting and Participants

Participants selected from an acute geriatric medical ward practicing CGA were part of a randomized control trial (RCT), registered at Clinical Trials (ID: NCT02773914), and approved by the Regional Ethical Review Board in Gothenburg (EPN Gothenburg Drn: 899-15). Ten participants aged 75 or older and screened as frail using the FRESH screen [24] were selected for this study. One month after discharge from the CGA ward, eight participants from the RCT were eligible for inclusion in the qualitative study if they scored a 25 or higher on the Mini Mental State (MMS) [25]. The remaining two participants who were not part of the RCT but received the CGA were declared cognitively intact by a physician on the ward and were contacted and asked if they were willing to be interviewed and recorded after one month after discharge from the CGA ward.

2.2. Data Collection

Ten individual, face-to-face interviews were conducted using open-ended questions which took place one month after discharge from the CGA ward. All participants signed informed consent forms and received both written and verbal information about the study prior to inclusion and being interviewed. All interviews were performed in the participant's home and were carried out from June 2016–May 2018 by the first author. The interviews were recorded digitally and lasted from 21 to 63 min. The research topics explored had the potential to be sensitive, and therefore the data collection was done individually in the comfort of the participant's home. Except for two of the participants who were interviewed at the same time as both had been admitted to the CGA ward and one of the participants who wanted their spouse to be present. The spouse contributed throughout the interview, complementing and enriching the participant's responses. Thus, in total ten participants aged 75–95 years were included: seven women and three men, as shown by the demographics in Table 1.

Table 1. Demographics of participants.

Participant	Age	Gender	Self Rated Health *	Living Status
#1	88	Male	Good	Married, lives with spouse
#2	85	Female	Good	Widow, lives alone
#3	92	Female	Fair	Widow, lives alone
#4	91	Female	Good	Widow, lives alone
#5	95	Female	Good	Widow, lives alone
#6**	86	Female	Fair	Married, lives with spouse
#7	77	Female	Very good	Divorced, lives alone
#8 ***	86	Male	Good	Married, lives with spouse
#9 ***	82	Female	Good	Married, lives with spouse
#10	91	Male	Poor	Widower, lives alone

* Self rated health: a single question taken from the Short-Form Health Survey (S-36) [26], asking: "How would you rate your health: excellent, very good, good, fair or poor" at one month follow-up. ** Spouse participated. ***Interviewed jointly with spouse (both were CGA recipients).

2.3. Data Analysis

Data was analyzed using conventional content analysis, following guidelines as described by Berg [23] and Hsieh [22]. In this analysis, the inquiry process focused on how the participants experienced being hospitalized, how they experienced they were treated, what services they received and how they experienced those services, and their goals and expectations while on the CGA ward. The analysis began with the observational processing of data, where the written data was read word by word, and exact words were then highlighted which seemed to capture key thoughts or concepts. Next, the researchers used these words to write notes about the thoughts and impressions gained from the data analysis. This process continued until labels for the codes began to emerge, which were reflective of groups of related thoughts. Code were then organized and sorted into categories to give the data meaning. The success of this analysis process relies heavily on the coding process which helps researchers to organize large amounts of text into fewer categories based on their content [27]. This inductive approach required researchers to shift their analytical directions, as the search for an emerging phenomenon was not based on people, objects, events, or situations by themselves [23], but rather was about the discovery of underlying meanings and content [22,28].

The first author—bilingual in English and Swedish—interviewed, recorded, transcribed, and translated verbatim all ten interviews from Swedish to English. Distinctive to using the conventional content analysis, researchers evaded using preconceived categories in their study and rather allowed the categories to be formed and named based on the emergence of data [22]. Frequent meetings were held by the researchers to analyze the findings; this further prompted that the emergent categories, subcategories, and codes could be defined and prepared as a written report where the findings were presented and then discussed related to previous research and the consequences related to the CGA phenomenon and process. Lastly, to strengthen trustworthiness when constructing and writing the report, data in the use of quotations from the frail older people were employed to strengthen the findings.

3. Results

3.1. Respected as a Person

Participants described how they were people with resources, previous knowledge, and carried with them their wants and wishes which made up their being as a person and feeling "respected as a person". Participants also described how they were ill patients in need of medical attention. The likelihood of feeling "respected as a person"—the core category identified in this study—explains how participants, despite being dependent on staff, experienced receiving attention while on a CGA ward. The staff's practices and behavior promoted participants feeling that they were welcomed, cared for, and respected. Participants wanted staff that were attentive, desired a confirmation of their existence, and to be ensured that they would receive help when it was needed. These experiences made them feel safe, calm, and valued, despite being ill on a medical ward. This was able to be achieved by having a reciprocal relationship with the ward staff which included engaging in communication and understanding while maintaining contact with each other on the ward. These experiences formed the category which was achieved by attentive staff that created an atmosphere and environment making up the category *participation in decision*-making. Feeling "respected as a person" is elucidated in Figure 1, visualizing the participants' experiences of receiving a comprehensive geriatric assessment on an acute geriatric ward.

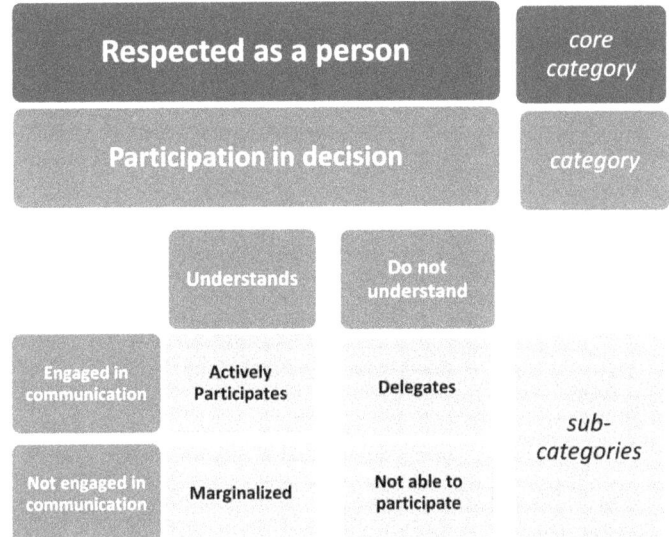

Figure 1. Experiences of receiving a comprehensive geriatric assessment visualized as a hierarchical process where participants felt; "respected as a person" (core category), when participation in decision (category) occurred while engaged in communication and able to understand, leading to four subcategories: actively participates, delegates, not able to participate, and marginalized.

3.2. Participation in Decision

Participation in decision emerged as the category which had to transpire on the ward if the participant was to achieve feeling "respected as a person". This process alluded to by the participants, focused on how their medical concerns were addressed by the ward staff who invited them to participate in decision-making related to their wants, wishes, and needs. Participation in decision-making required that the participant engaged in communication with the staff and were able to achieve an understanding of their own situation. When engaged in communication, the participants experienced favorable attention or interest from staff while sharing and receiving information on the CGA ward. Understanding was also required if the participants were to comprehend what was happening to them on the CGA ward. Understanding could also be experienced as a reciprocal relationship, which was achieved between the participants and the staff. Participants' understanding of their situation, medical status, treatment, ward routines, discharge plans, and the way in which they processed their experienced circumstances could vary depending on how ill they were while on the ward. Furthermore, it also depended on how they experienced how they were approached by the staff working on the ward and if they were invited to participate in decision-making. Frail older people's perceptions of participation in decision-making was expressed from four dimensions: actively participates, delegates, not able to participate, and marginalized, as shown in Figure 1.

3.3. Actively Participates

When a participant was *actively participating* in decision-making, it necessitated that they were included, which required that they understood their situation, such as medical status, treatment, ward routines, and discharge plans. It also required that they were engaged in communication with the staff so that information could be exchanged and understood, which allowed them to reach a decision together with the CGA staff. One man described how he and his wife experienced actively participating in the decision-making process prior to being discharged home from the ward.

#8 "They asked and you could tell them what you were thinking or what you needed help with they said you can have help with this and that, and we said no we want to have help with this and that. It felt like they listened to us, and then we made a decision."

Another aspect of the actively participating experience was described by one woman who humbly described how she did not initially see or understand what the staff did. They took the time to share their knowledge, information, and concerns to improve her understanding prior to the decision-making process.

#3 "They understood that I needed additional treatment. I didn't understand that myself. A stubborn old lady who thinks I am going to manage myself ... so I had a bit of education ... I got treatment and they discovered what I needed."

3.4. Delegates

When a participant was engaged in communication but did not experience that they understood the situation enough for their *participation in decision*-making, their decision was to delegate. While the participant was engaged in communication with the staff, they chose to authorize the staff on the ward to act or represent them in a situation which required that a decision be made. Thus, the decision made by the participant was deliberate, as they were informed and understood what they were consenting to by deciding not to participate. This occurred when participants felt that the staff had better knowledge and understanding of the medical situation, so they delegated the decision-making to the staff.

When participants perceived that the staff understood, were empathetic, competent, and/or action driven, it could result in them offering suggestions and solutions to make the situation more safe or comfortable. One woman highlighted her call for help, as she communicated her concern to the staff, eluding to the importance of the staff listening skills and understanding her acute medical needs, where she delegated the responsibility to the staff.

#6 "I told them I was going to jump from the 8th floor and die and the doctor spoke with [husband] ... and said we need to do something".

3.5. Not Able to Participate

When a participant was not engaged in communication and did not understand because they felt too ill, or because the staff determined that a patient was not able to participate due to being too ill, then the staff made decisions without consulting or informing the participant. This usually occurred in the early stages of the acute medical treatment, when participants were not alert or cognizant, and participants accepted this as a necessary part of their care. One woman described her experience of being very ill when she arrived to the CGA ward after a difficult experience in the emergency department, where she did not need to decide anything.

#4 "I was a bit confused during that time, but they told me at the hospital I was lying on ward X ... they took tests every morning ... and I received lots of antibiotics in an IV."

If a participant did not experience a joint consensus with the staff founded on communication and understanding, the likelihood of participating in decision-making and feeling "respected as a person" was diminished. Understanding while dependent on a person's resources and previous knowledge is also heavily weighed on the approach used by the other person. If a participant did not understand, and the staff did not make an effort to share their information and insight with the other person, then an ignorant, ill-informed position is likely to result. One man who acknowledged that despite not comprehending why he was admitted to the hospital, he did not ask the staff to explain his situation.

#10 "When one is in the hospital, there are some things as a person that you don't really understand."

Participants described how they could lack receiving verbal information and thus not being able to understand their situation. One woman expressed how important engagement in communication was for them and how they looked forward to experiencing that the staff would take a personal interest and give them the attention they so desired prior to discharge.

#6 "There was supposed to be a meeting, but it never happened. The doctor at the hospital said ... that we would have a meeting ... but it didn't happen ... the doctor is poor at explaining possibilities. They don't say it directly, we can't heal that. Instead they go the side and start talking about something else ... so it is just left lying there".

However, she reported receiving a written form of communication at discharge. This written information was not preferred if it was experienced as replacing a conversation. However, a written form of communication was welcomed by participants who wanted it as a complement clarifying the information verbally shared. #6 "A plan of care from the doctor ... we got that when we were going home ... what had happened, which medicine was prescribed ... they were going to follow up with me at the clinic ... which is good."

3.6. Marginalized

A participant was marginalized from participation in decision-making when not engaged in communication, informed, or given the privilege to know what was going on, despite their ability to understand. When participants became aware that they were excluded or marginalized from participation in decisions, as the staff on the ward had made decisions for the participant, it could be related to their medical concerns or the organizational routines on the ward. However, participants did not want to complain or bother staff with small things, as was the case of one participant who changed room three times in four days and described how it was to share a room with a patient with dementia who woke them during the night caressing their arm. However, feeling marginalized from the organizational routines prevented them from reporting it or complaining to the staff, despite the fact that their personal space was not respected by a fellow patient.

#9 "It was a bit strange ... but we didn't question their decision [regarding room organization]; we figured they had enough to do."

Another marginalized episode can be illustrated when the participant experienced that the shared information they exchanged with the staff was not acknowledged or received, or when the staff gave them information but there was no opportunity to discuss. A unidirectional communication method resulted in the participants feeling that there was disengagement with the ward staff; due to a lack of information, which made them unaware of their medical status and conditions or what was expected of them. This in turn could affect future issues related to the participant's medications, treatments, symptoms, or discharge plans. One woman expressed how sudden and impersonal the decision that was made on her behalf without her knowledge was experienced when the staff told her she had to change hospitals:

#4 "They just came in and told me I was moving ... it happened very fast."

Lastly, experiences of being marginalized occurred when an engaging conversation was neglected and resulted in the staff's lack of understanding related to patients' care, treatment, and medication while on the ward. One participant described how she felt that she had information that the staff did not understand or acknowledge, which caused her to be misdiagnosed and mistreated.

#2 "They filled me with very strong medicine ... even morphine for the pain ... I wasn't admitted for pain. They should have understood that something was wrong, instead of giving me loads of painkillers. I was admitted for vertigo."

4. Discussion

This study is among the few to have used qualitative interviews to ascertain frail older people's experiences of receiving a comprehensive geriatric assessment on an acute geriatric ward. Participants who felt that they were welcome and cared for by attentive staff, who confirmed their existence as a person, was what frail older people in this study described. This experience was strengthened by the person-centered approach used by staff on the CGA ward which made them feel "respected as a person". Ekman et al. [29] found that when staff practiced person-centered care the person felt placed at the center of their clinical decisions, which considered their strengths, future plans, and rights.

Person-centered care is critical for ensuring quality geriatric medical and health care services, and person-centered care is law in Sweden; Patient Act (2014:821) [30] which states that patients should be treated as people who participate in decision-making.

The positive experiences of frail older people when included to *participate in decision*-making in this study resulted in participants feeling "respected as a person". They also experienced this when the staff practiced approaches which enabled their engagement and participation in decisions. Ringdal et al. [31] found that participation is best promoted on the ward and that it begins with the team's understanding of the participant's unique needs for care and their preferences, where establishing a good relationship with patients and understanding their ability to participate despite medical concerns is beneficial. The quality of interactions of older people's experiences with ward staff explored by Bridges et al. [32] reported that experiences were shaped by how their hospital admission was perceived. This primarily was related to how they wanted the staff to interact with them so they could maintain their identity ("see who I am"), create community ("connect with me"), and share decision-making ("involve me") [32]. The results in our study strongly concur and correlate with Bridges [32], as the framework concept development generated in this study found. Our study's participants experienced and felt "respected as a person"; the "see who I am" felt engaged in communication and understood; the "connect with me" and included to participate in decision-making; the "involve me" when staff practiced person-centered care on the CGA ward. In this context, a previous study [31] found that it is beneficial to establish a good relationship with patients and an understanding of their ability to participate, despite their medical concerns. Similarly, Chawla et al. [33] suggested that the approaches used by staff must be nuanced and encourage patients to participate in decision-making in ways they are most comfortable. Reasons to include patients to participate reported by Eldh et al. [34] found that patients continued to experience that they were self-reliant, comprehended the situation, and maintained a sense of control when included.

In this study, frail older people's experiences of an acute geriatric ward practicing CGA are highlighted as a complex and dynamic phenomenon, and that they did not always experience as person-centered care. Obstacles which arose hindering person-centered care from systematically occurring were identified when participants in this study experienced that when they were too ill and the staff did not involve them to participate in decisions related to their care. However, such an approach must be considered viable; as these participants were not avoided or discouraged from participating in making decisions after being informed. Rather they were limited in their cognitive capacities, restricting and preventing optimal communication and understanding, which was clinically assessed by the ward staff. Therefore, the term to describe the care they received is not a person-centered approach, but rather an alternative term of "person-supportive care" as suggested by Entwistle et al. [35]. According to Munthe et al. [36], person-centered care is intended to empower and liberate patients. However, when a person is dependent, vulnerable, or fragile, these practices are challenged. In this case, practicing shared decision-making with people meeting the criteria described by Munthe et al. [36] may have an adverse effect, which leads to disempowering, exploiting, and even harming the person it was intended to support. Therefore, it can be reasoned, as in the case of this study, that frail older people not included in decision-making due to their cognitively frail state were still cared for and supported by staff with competence and understanding, but they were not empowered to make decisions when their capabilities were limited.

In this study when participants experienced not feeling "respected as a person", they expressed that these failures or shortcomings may have been due to the ward's organizational structure, staff behavior, and/or staffing issues, which limited or hindered practicing person-centered care being practiced on the CGA ward. A CGA should be used to assess, treat, and plan future care with frail older people [8,37,38]. Entwistle et al. [35] found that staff must understand patient goals and capabilities, despite the fact that medical and health care policies may occasionally promote initiatives that overlook that patients are people. An earlier study warned health professionals [38] that if they do not understand patient preferences, overlook or misinterpret the person, the consequences could be as harmful as misdiagnosing a disease. McCormack et al. [19] advises person-centered care is best achieved by staff who are knowledgeable and competent in practicing the approach. However, Steward et al. [39] states that learning the practices of a person-centered care approach are challenging, time consuming, and take effort to learn the professional skills and competency required for mastering this approach. Ekman [29,40] highlights that person-centeredness requires funding and supportive government directives to secure the necessary training and organizational practices needed on the hospital ward are given priority.

Participants in this study, when experiencing that the staff did not communicate with them, did not take time to understand them, and/or did not include them in making decisions; person-centered care was not being practiced. This was most likely due to traditional practices and professional attitudes which dictated how services were provided, creating organizational barriers in health care delivery as identified in earlier studies [41,42]. By further developing and supporting the organizational practices and policies on a CGA ward, gaps could be discovered as to why patient-centered care was not always experienced by the frail older people receiving the care. Therefore, CGA could benefit from including a patient satisfaction survey, such as the Hospital Consumer Assessment of Healthcare Providers and Systems survey [43] (HCAHPS survey) or the Swedish National Patient Survey [44], as a part of their comprehensive assessment after discharge. This would allow the team practicing person-centered care to have insight and feedback about patients' perspectives related to their care. Access to data and information identified as important to the recipients of a CGA would better enable staff to learn of their shortcomings and work towards making continuous improvements related to the quality of care they provide to frail older people. By making these survey reports public, an increase in accountability and transparency could influence other medical wards not practicing CGA and person-centered care to strive to increase patient satisfaction when treating frail older people. Therefore, measuring patient-perceived quality and experiences of health care and participation in future studies with frail older people could be useful to improve and further develop the health care system from a marginalized patient's perspective.

Methodological Considerations and Limitations

Employing a secondary analysis was deemed feasible as the researchers' intent was to perform a more in-depth analysis of the findings discovered in the initial study with a subset of data from that study [45]. In the case of this study, a secondary analysis of data from the initial study was used to understand the experiences of receiving a CGA, as this appeared important but was not sufficiently concentrated on in the first analysis. Trustworthiness of qualitative studies founded on secondary data analysis may be viewed as less credible because of the relationship between the researchers and the data set [45]. However, in the case of this study, the interviews, transcriptions, and analysis of data in the initial study were performed by the first author. According to Hinds et al. [45], with this closeness to data comes benefits related to the context of the study. On the contrary, the closeness may also lead researchers to prematurely establish an understanding of the phenomenon that was present in the data set but was not the focus of the initial study [45]. Aware of these concerns, the researchers closely followed the conventional content analysis method guidelines and the phenomenon which emerged was not based on preconceptions or findings of the initial study but rather surfaced as the latent meanings and content verbalized during the interviews. Additional limitations to this study are that the sample was small, taken from a native Swedish population, which was primarily women with mild to good cognitive capacity. Future studies would benefit from using a larger sample of internationally diverse participants with less cognitive capacity and a better female-to-male ratio, so that the concept development of feeling "respected as a person" could be further explored with greater diversity when being compared with this study's findings.

5. Conclusions

Receiving a comprehensive geriatric assessment when including person-centered care made the frail older patient feel "respected as a person" despite being a patient. However, if a person-centered care approach does not work because the person is too ill to participate, then care must be delivered as person-supportive care. Conversely, when a person-centered care approach is not practiced, the consequences are that patients despite a CGA model may be hindered from feeling "respected as a person". Therefore, a CGA could benefit from the use of a patient satisfaction survey after discharge to better understand the health care gaps experienced from a patient's perspective.

Author Contributions: T.W. is a PhD student, researcher, collected the data, transcribed the data, and drafted the manuscript. T.W., I.O.H., K.W., and S.D.I. are responsible for the study design, and reviewed and edited the manuscript. All authors have read and approved the submitted version of the manuscript.

Funding: This research was supported financially by FORTE (diary number 2015-00043), Region Västra Götaland (ALFGRG-530971 and VGFOUREG-565511) and The Kind Gustav and Queen Victoria Freemasons Foundation. The funders took no part in the design or execution of the study.

Acknowledgments: Special thanks to the care coordinators at Sahlgrenska University Hospital for their participation in patient inclusion.

Ethical approval: All subjects gave their informed consent for inclusion before they participated in the study. The study was conducted in accordance with the Declaration of Helsinki, and ethical approval is confirmed (EPN Gbg dn4 899-15).

Conflicts of Interest: The authors declare that they have no competing interests.

References

1. Health Care in Sweden. Available online: https://sweden.se/society/health-care-in-sweden/ (accessed on 23 January 2019).
2. Ekerstad, N.; Karlson, B.W.; Dahlin Ivanoff, S.; Landahl, S.; Andersson, D.; Heintz, E.; Husberg, M.; Alwin, J. Is the acute care of frail elderly patients in a comprehensive geriatric assessment unit superior to conventional acute medical care? *Clin. Interv. Aging* **2017**, *12*, 1–9. [CrossRef] [PubMed]
3. Ferrucci, L.; Guralnik, J.M.; Studenski, S.; Fried, L.P.; Cutler, G.B., Jr.; Walston, J.D. Designing randomized, controlled trials aimed at preventing or delaying functional decline and disability in frail, older persons: A consensus report. *J. Am. Geriatr. Soc.* **2004**, *52*, 625–634. [CrossRef] [PubMed]
4. Gill, T.M.; Baker, D.I.; Gottschalk, M.; Peduzzi, P.N.; Allore, H.; Byers, A. A program to prevent functional decline in physically frail, elderly persons who live at home. *N. Engl. J. Med.* **2002**, *347*, 1068–1074. [CrossRef] [PubMed]
5. Gill, T.M. Education, prevention, and the translation of research into practice. *J. Am. Geriatr. Soc.* **2005**, *53*, 724–726. [CrossRef] [PubMed]
6. Fried, L.P.; Ferrucci, L.; Darer, J.; Williamson, J.D.; Anderson, G. Untangling the concepts of disability, frailty, and comorbidity: Implications for improved targeting and care. *J. Gerontol. Ser. A Biol. Sci. Med. Sci.* **2004**, *59*, 255–263. [CrossRef]
7. Rockwood, K. What would make a definition of frailty successful? *Age Ageing* **2005**, *34*, 432–434. [CrossRef]
8. Ward, K.T.; Reuben, D.B. Comprehensive Geriatric Assessment. Available online: https://www.uptodate.com/contents/comprehensive-geriatric-assessment (accessed on 8 March 2018).
9. Singer, S.J.; Burgers, J.; Friedberg, M.; Rosenthal, M.B.; Leape, L.; Schneider, E. Defining and measuring integrated patient care: Promoting the next frontier in health care delivery. *Med. Care Res. Rev.* **2011**, *68*, 112–127. [CrossRef]
10. Duner, A.; Blomberg, S.; Hasson, H. Implementing a continuum of care model for older people-results from a Swedish case study. *Int. J. Integr. Care* **2011**, *11*, e136. [CrossRef]
11. Rubenstein, L.Z.; Siu, A.L.; Wieland, D. Comprehensive geriatric assessment: Toward understanding its efficacy. *Aging Clin. Exp. Res.* **1989**, *1*, 87–98. [CrossRef]
12. World Health Organization. WHO, Active Aging: A Policy Framework. Available online: https://www.who.int/ageing/publications/active_ageing/en/ (accessed on 19 September 2018).

13. Westgard, T.; Ottenvall Hammar, I.; Holmgren, E.; Ehrenberg, A.; Wisten, A.; Ekdahl, A.W.; Dahlin-Ivanoff, S.; Wilhelmson, K. Comprehensive geriatric assessment pilot of a randomized control study in a Swedish acute hospital: A feasibility study. *Pilot Feasibility Stud.* **2018**, *4*, 41. [CrossRef]
14. Ellis, G.; Gardner, M.; Tsiachristas, A.; Langhorne, P.; Burke, O.; Harwood, R.H.; Conroy, S.P.; Kircher, T.; Somme, D.; Saltvedt, I.; et al. Comprehensive geriatric assessment for older adults admitted to hospital. *Cochrane Database Syst. Rev.* **2017**, *9*, CD006211. [CrossRef] [PubMed]
15. Aberg, A.C.; Ehrenberg, A. Inpatient geriatric care in Sweden-Important factors from an inter-disciplinary team perspective. *Arch. Gerontol. Geriatr.* **2017**, *72*, 113–120. [CrossRef]
16. Morgan, J.H. On Becoming a Person (1961) Carl Rogers' Celebrated Classic in Memorian. *J. Psychol. Issues Organ. Cult.* **2011**, *2*, 95–105. [CrossRef]
17. Leplege, A.; Gzil, F.; Cammelli, M.; Lefeve, C.; Pachoud, B.; Ville, I. Person-centredness: Conceptual and historical perspectives. *Disabil. Rehabil.* **2007**, *29*, 1555–1565. [CrossRef] [PubMed]
18. Kitwood, T. On being a person. In *Dementia Reconsidered: The Person Comes First*; Kitwood, T., Ed.; Open University Press: Philadelphia, PA, USA, 1997; pp. 7–19.
19. McCormack, B.; McCance, T.V. Development of a framework for person-centred nursing. *J. Adv. Nurs.* **2006**, *56*, 472–479. [CrossRef] [PubMed]
20. Esbensen, B.A.; Hvitved, I.; Andersen, H.E.; Petersen, C.M. Growing older in the context of needing geriatric assessment: A qualitative study. *Scand. J. Caring Sci.* **2016**, *30*, 489–498. [CrossRef] [PubMed]
21. Darby, J.; Williamson, T.; Logan, P.; Gladman, J. Comprehensive geriatric assessment on an acute medical unit: A qualitative study of older people's and informal carer's perspectives of the care and treatment received. *Clin. Rehabil.* **2017**, *31*, 126–134. [CrossRef]
22. Hsieh, H.F.; Shannon, S.E. Three approaches to qualitative content analysis. *Qual. Health Res.* **2005**, *15*, 1277–1288. [CrossRef] [PubMed]
23. Berg, B. *Qualitative Research Methods for the Social Scineces*, 6th ed.; Pearson Education, Inc.: Boston, MA, USA, 2007.
24. Kajsa, E.; Katarina, W.; Sten, L.; Synneve, I.D. Screening for frailty among older emergency department visitors: Validation of the new FRESH-screening instrument. *BMC Emerg. Med.* **2016**, *16*, 27. [CrossRef]
25. Folstein, M.F.; Folstein, S.E.; McHugh, P.R. "Mini-mental state". A practical method for grading the cognitive state of patients for the clinician. *J. Psychiatr. Res.* **1975**, *12*, 189–198. [CrossRef]
26. Ware, J.E., Jr.; Sherbourne, C.D. The MOS 36-item short-form health survey (SF-36). I. Conceptual framework and item selection. *Med. Care* **1992**, *30*, 473–483. [CrossRef] [PubMed]
27. Weber, R.P. *Basic Content Analysis*, 2nd ed.; Sage: Beverly Hills, CA, USA, 1990.
28. Kondracki, N.L.; Wellman, N.S.; Amundson, D.R. Content analysis: Review of methods and their applications in nutrition education. *J. Nutr. Educ. Behav.* **2002**, *34*, 224–230. [CrossRef]
29. Ekman, I.; Swedberg, K.; Taft, C.; Lindseth, A.; Norberg, A.; Brink, E.; Carlsson, J.; Dahlin-Ivanoff, S.; Johansson, I.L.; Kjellgren, K.; et al. Person-centered care—Ready for prime time. *Eur. J. Cardiovasc. Nurs.* **2011**, *10*, 248–251. [CrossRef] [PubMed]
30. Sveriges Riksdag. The Patient Act (2014:821). Available online: https://www.riksdagen.se/sv/dokument-lagar/dokument/svensk-forfattningssamling/patientlag-2014821_sfs-2014-821/ (accessed on 24 January 2019).
31. Ringdal, M.; Chaboyer, W.; Ulin, K.; Bucknall, T.; Oxelmark, L. Patient preferences for participation in patient care and safety activities in hospitals. *BMC Nurs.* **2017**, *16*, 69. [CrossRef] [PubMed]
32. Bridges, J.; Flatley, M.; Meyer, J. Older people's and relatives' experiences in acute care settings: Systematic review and synthesis of qualitative studies. *Int. J. Nurs. Stud.* **2010**, *47*, 89–107. [CrossRef]
33. Chawla, N.; Arora, N.K. Why do some patients prefer to leave decisions up to the doctor: Lack of self-efficacy or a matter of trust? *J. Cancer Surviv. Res. Pract.* **2013**, *7*, 592–601. [CrossRef] [PubMed]
34. Eldh, A.C.; Ehnfors, M.; Ekman, I. The phenomena of participation and non-participation in health care—Experiences of patients attending a nurse-led clinic for chronic heart failure. *Eur. J. Cardiovasc. Nurs.* **2004**, *3*, 239–246. [CrossRef]
35. Entwistle, V.A.; Watt, I.S. A Capabilities Approach to Person-Centered Care: Response to Open Peer Commentaries on "Treating Patients as Persons: A Capabilities Approach to Support Delivery of Person-Centered Care". *Am. J. Bioeth.* **2013**, *13*, W1–W4. [CrossRef]

36. Munthe, C.; El-Alti, L.; Hartvigsson, T.; Nijsingh, N. Disputing with patients in person-centered care: Ethical aspects in standard care, pediatrics, psychiatry and public health. *J. Argum. Context* **2018**, *7*, 231–244. [CrossRef]
37. Ellis, G.; Whitehead, M.A.; Robinson, D.; O'Neill, D.; Langhorne, P. Comprehensive geriatric assessment for older adults admitted to hospital: Meta-analysis of randomised controlled trials. *BMJ (Clin. Res. Ed.)* **2011**, *343*, d6553. [CrossRef]
38. Mulley, A.G.; Trimble, C.; Elwyn, G. Stop the silent misdiagnosis: Patients' preferences matter. *BMJ (Clin. Res. Ed.)* **2012**, *345*, e6572. [CrossRef] [PubMed]
39. Steward, M.; Brown, B.J.; Weston, W.W.; McWhinney, I.R.; McWilliam, C.L.; Freeman, T.R. *Patient-Centered Medicine Transforming the Clinical Method*, 2nd ed.; Radcliffe Medical Press: Oxon, UK, 2006.
40. Ekman, I.; Hedman, H.; Swedberg, K.; Wallengren, C. Commentary: Swedish initiative on person centred care. *BMJ (Clin. Res. Ed.)* **2015**, *350*, h160. [CrossRef] [PubMed]
41. Mareš, J. People-centred health care: A good idea but difficult to implement. *Kontakt* **2017**, *1*, 1–3. [CrossRef]
42. Moore, L.; Britten, N.; Lydahl, D.; Naldemirci, O.; Elam, M.; Wolf, A. Barriers and facilitators to the implementation of person-centred care in different healthcare contexts. *Scand. J. Caring Sci.* **2017**, *31*, 662–673. [CrossRef] [PubMed]
43. Center for Medicare & Medicaid Services. Hospital Consumer Assessment of Healthcare Providers and Systems urvey. Available online: https://www.cms.gov/Medicare/Quality-Initiatives-Patient-Assessment-instruments/hospitalqualityinits/hospitalHCAHPS.html (accessed on 10 January 2019).
44. Sveriges Landsting och Regioner I Samverkan. National Patient Survey. Available online: https://patientenkat.se/sv/english/ (accessed on 10 January 2019).
45. Hinds, P.; Vogel, R.J.; Clarke-Steffan, L. The possibilities and pitfalls of doing a secondary analysis of a qualitative data set. *Qual. Health Res.* **1997**, *7*, 408–424. [CrossRef]

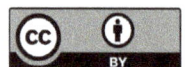

© 2019 by the authors. Licensee MDPI, Basel, Switzerland. This article is an open access article distributed under the terms and conditions of the Creative Commons Attribution (CC BY) license (http://creativecommons.org/licenses/by/4.0/).

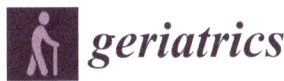

Article

The Relationship of Balance Disorders with Falling, the Effect of Health Problems, and Social Life on Postural Balance in the Elderly Living in a District in Turkey

Tahsin Barış Değer [1,*], Zeliha Fulden Saraç [2], Emine Sumru Savaş [2] and Selahattin Fehmi Akçiçek [2]

1. Directorate of Health Affairs, Söke Municipality, Söke, Aydın 09200, Turkey
2. Geriatrics Section, Faculty of Medicine, Ege University, Bornova, Izmir 35100, Turkey; fulden.sarac@ege.edu.tr (Z.F.S.); emine.sumru.savas@ege.edu.tr (E.S.S.); fehmi.akcicek@gmail.com (S.F.A.)
* Correspondence: baris.deger@soke.bel.tr; Tel.: +90-542-3233854

Received: 11 March 2019; Accepted: 15 May 2019; Published: 17 May 2019

Abstract: The aim of this study was to determine the prevalence of balance disorders; the effects of sociodemographic, medical, and social conditions on postural balance; and the relationship between balance and falls in elderly individuals. The study design was cross-sectional. A total of 607 community-dwelling elderly individuals with a mean age of 73.99 ± 6.6 years were enrolled after being selected by stratified random sampling. The study was performed as a face-to-face survey in the homes of elderly individuals. Sociodemographic and medical data were obtained from elderly individuals using the Elderly Identification Form. Balance disorders were determined using the Berg Balance Scale (BBS). In this study, the prevalence of balance disorders was found to be 34.3% in the community-dwelling elderly. Older age, physical disability, having four or more chronic illnesses, the presence of incontinence, having a history of falls, not walking regularly, absence of free time activity, and obesity were found to be associated with an increased prevalence of balance disorders. Balance disorders are commonly seen in the elderly and may be triggered by a variety of biological and social factors. It is crucial to develop and implement national health and social policies to eliminate the causes of this problem, as well as to prioritize preventive health services in the ever-increasing elderly population.

Keywords: balance disorder; prevalence; elderly; fall; medical conditions; social mobility

1. Introduction

Balance is the ability to collect sensory and proprioceptive signals related to a person's position in space and to produce the appropriate motor responses to control body movement [1]. When this ability deteriorates, due to both disease and the normal aging process, the risk of falling increases in the elderly [2]. Balance disorders are one of the most important reasons leading to falls [3]. Falling increases the possibility of death and disability; furthermore, it may cause the loss of independence [4]. In 2014, an estimated 29 million falls were reported in the US. Twenty-seven thousand older adults died, and 7 million were injured because of falls [5]. Approximately 68% of hospitalizations of injured elderly individuals were reported to be because of falls, and this rate reached 86% in individuals aged ≥85 years [6]. Falls in the elderly population cause long-term immobilization and related complications. Therefore, balance disorders in elderly individuals are a symptom that leads to functional insufficiency. As a result of dynamic postural control, appropriate rehabilitation following the early detection of balance disorders and environmental modifications could prevent falls and increase an individual's quality of life [7].

Balance disorders generate a significant healthcare burden due to the rise in hospitalization, morbidities, and mortalities in the elderly population [8]. Most of the patients who present to emergency services complain of balance disorders. In otology and neurology clinics, in which patients commonly present with balance disorders and dizziness, the rate of balance disorder is about 20% [9]. Thirteen percent of community-dwelling individuals aged 65–69 years and 46% of those aged ≥85 years have balance disorders [10]. There are many factors that lead to balance disorders, including cardiovascular diseases, metabolic diseases, musculoskeletal disorders, neurological disorders, visual and hearing disturbance, fear of falling, surgical operations, and specific medications [11].

Factors related to the risk of falling were taken into consideration in a report published by the World Health Organization (WHO) on the elderly in 2007. It was reported that balance disorders contribute to the occurrence of falls, and that balance exercises are a useful way to protect from falls. [12]. Goal number three of the Turkey Healthy Aging Implementation Program in the Healthy Aging Action Plan and Implementation Program published by the Ministry of Health for 2015–2020 includes a statement on the development of preventive and rehabilitative approaches to determine and decrease the risk factors leading to balance disorders, falling, and fear of falling in old age [13].

This study was conducted to determine the prevalence of balance disorders in the elderly population, identify the health (chronic illnesses, drug use) and social (leisure time activities) causes of balance disorders, and determine the role of balance disorders in falls.

2. Materials and Methods

2.1. Subjects

This was a cross-sectional study involving community-dwelling elderly individuals aged >65 years in a center in the Söke district of Aydın. A total of 607 elderly individuals with a mean age of 73.99 ± 6.6 (65–102) years were selected by the stratified random sampling method. The 65–74-year age group was stratified as the first group, the 75–84-year age group was the second group, and the ≥85-year age group was the third group. The study was performed as face-to-face surveys at the homes of elderly individuals. A total of 668 elderly individuals were asked to participate in the study, but those individuals who were bedridden, who were diagnosed with dementia, and who did not pass the Mini Mental State Examination (MMSE; cut-off score of 23) were not included in the study [14]. Eventually, 607 elderly individuals who agreed to voluntarily participate in the study formed the sample used for our study. Informed consent was given by all participants.

2.2. Evaluation Parameters

Elderly Identification Form: This form recorded information about the participants, including their age, gender, marital status, number of people in their household, economic level, education level, presence of illnesses, disability status, fall history, fear of falling, drugs used, presence of incontinence, nocturia, walking habits, leisure time activities, and body mass index. This form was created by the investigators.

Berg Balance Scale (BBS): This test, which was developed to measure balance performance in elderly individuals, consists of 14 instructions. Participants are given 0–4 points for each instruction according to their ability to perform the task; the maximum total score for the test is 56. It is a practical test that can be conducted in 15–20 min in the homes of the community-dwelling elderly individuals. The cut-off score for the test is 45. A score of 45–56 is an indication of an acceptable functional level. A score below 45 point is considered to indicate a balance disorder [15–17]. The Turkish translation and the transcultural adaptation of the BBS were previously studied in 60 elderly individuals with various comorbidities aged >65 years, and the validity and reliability have been reported [18].

2.3. Methods

The study started with the selection of Address-Based Population Registration System data with a stratified random sampling method for individuals over 65 years of age. The elders who were selected by this method represented elderly people living in the district center. Thus, the sample used was representative of the group of universe of elderly people in the district center. Four different teams were formed in the study, and these teams visited the elderly in their homes. The MMSE was applied to elderly people who participated voluntarily, who were not bedridden, and who had not been diagnosed with dementia. The Elderly Identification Form was given to participants to determine their socio-demographic and health characteristics, as well as to gather information about their free life activities. Sociodemographic, social, and health data were recorded on the form. Participants' health reports were reviewed. The drugs they used were noted. The participants completed the BBS assessment, and their BBS scores were noted. The weights and heights of the participants were measured, and BMI values were calculated.

The present study was submitted to and approved by the Clinical Research Ethics Committee of the Ege University Faculty of Medicine (Decision Number: 16–3.2/7, Date: April 7, 2016). The study was conducted in accordance with the Declaration of Helsinki. All participants provided informed consent before being included in the study as a participant.

2.4. Statistics

Analysis of the data was done using SPSS (Version 18.0, SPSS Inc., Chicago, IL, USA). Chi-square tests were used to analyze balance disorders and fall variables. Univariate binary logistic regression analysis and multiple binary logistic regression analyses were conducted on all variables. For the results of the statistical analysis, p-values of <0.05 were considered significant.

3. Results

3.1. The Prevalence of Balance Disorders (Mean Value of BBS)

The BBS was used to measure the prevalence of balance disorders in the participants. In elderly individuals, the cut-off (sorter) value for balance disorders is 45 points [19,20]. The prevalence of a balance disorder in the elderly individuals in our study was 34.3%. The average BBS score was 43.49 ± 14.2.

3.2. The Relationship between Balance and Falls

For individuals with a balance disorder, 58.1% had fallen in the past year, and 90.3% had a fear of falling; in those without a balance disorder, 29.8% had fallen, and 60.3% had a fear of falling (Table 1).

Table 1. The relationship between balance and falling.

	Fell Last Year			Fear of Falling		
	Yes (n = 237)	No (n = 370)	Chi-square (p-value)	Yes (n = 427)	No (n = 178)	Chi-square (p-value)
Balance disorder (n = 208)	121 (58.1%)	87 (41.8%)	$X^2 = (p < 0.001)$	187 (90.3%)	20 (9.7%)	$X^2 = (p < 0.001)$
No balance disorder (n = 389)	116 (29.8%)	283 (72.7%)		240 (60.3%)	158 (39.7%)	

Chi-square test, $p < 0.05$: statistically significant.

3.3. Multiple Logistic Regression Analysis and the Effects of Sociodemographic, Medical, and Social Data on Balance Disorders

The sample of 607 participants was composed of 347 people aged 65–74 (first group), 214 aged 75–84 (second group), and 46 aged over 85 years old (third group). The association of age with balance disorders was statistically significant according to the multiple logistic regression analysis ($p = 0.002$).

The prevalence of balance disorders increased as age increased. Balance disorders were 1.97 times higher in the second group ($p = 0.006$, OR = 1.97, 95% CI = 1.21–3.20) and 3.63 times higher in the third group ($p = 0.003$, OR = 3.63, 95% CI = 1.54–8.55), compared with the first group.

Three hundred and sixty-one of the 607 participants (59.47%) were females.

Participants included non-literate individuals, primary school quitters, primary school graduates (n = 276), secondary school graduates, high school graduates, and university graduates.

Participants included widows (divorced or had lost their husband/wife) and married individuals.

Participants included those living alone, with their spouses, with their spouses and children, only with their children, and with relatives/carers.

Considering economic situations, there were people without incomes, those receiving the elderly/widow/disabled wage, those receiving the retirement wage, and those using wages earned by their spouse.

The variables gender, education level, marital status, living status, and economic situation were not found to be statistically significant in our study, according to the multiple logistic regression analysis.

Our study included elderly participants without any obstacles, elderly participants with a visual impairment, elderly participants with a hearing impairment, and elderly participants with disabilities. When the relationship between the disability status of elderly people and balance disorders was examined, with the group without obstacles taken as the reference group, participants with walking disabilities had a balance disorder 2.80 times higher than the reference group ($p = 0.013$, OR = 2.80, 95% CI = 1.24–6.33). The disability variable was found to be statistically significant (Table 2).

Two hundred and thirty-seven participants had fallen at least once in the past year. Fall history was statistically associated with the presence of a balance disorder in our study, according to the multiple logistic regression analysis. The prevalence of balance disorders among those who had fallen in the past year was 2.25 times higher than in those who had not fallen ($p < 0.001$, OR = 2.25, 95% CI = 1.46–3.46).

The prevalence of chronic disease was determined. Only 10.7% (n = 65) of the participants did not have any chronic illnesses. The number of chronic diseases was not statistically significantly associated with the prevalence of balance disorders in our study, according to multiple logistic regression analysis, but a significant association was shown in elderly people with four or more diseases ($p = 0.047$, OR = 3.54, 95% CI = 1.01–12.32).

Daily medication use was recorded for each participant. Hundreds of medications were classified according to their indications to determine which drugs can alter balance. For example, a participant using three medications (amlodipine [a selective calcium channel blocker], silazapril and hydrochlorothiazide [an angiotensin-converting enzyme inhibitor combination], and acetylsalicylic acid [an antithrombotic agent]) was categorized into a group of participants "using only one group of medications" (cardiovascular drug group). Medications were determined by group number instead of individual drugs. Our study included participants using neurological disease drugs, cardiovascular group drugs, diabetes medications, vertigo medications, thyroid medications, rheumatic disease drugs, pain killers, and depression group drugs. 12.8% of the participants (n = 78) did not use any medication (Table 2). The drug group use variable was not shown to be significantly associated with balance disorders in our study.

One hundred and seventy-seven of the participants stated that they could not hold urine during the day. In addition, 87 of the participants stated that they could not hold urine sometimes. Urinary incontinence was found to be statistically significantly associated with balance disorders ($p = 0.002$). Compared with the participants who had no difficulty with urinary incontinence, balance disorders were 2.4 times more prevalent in the participants who had urinary incontinence ($p = 0.001$, OR = 2.4, 95%CI = 1.46–3.95).

Table 2. Univariate logistic regression analysis and multiple logistic regression analysis.

Variant	Reference Group (n)	Other Groups (n)	Univariate Logistic Regression			** Multiple Logistic Regression		
			P	OR	95% C.I.	P	OR	95% C.I.
Age						0.002 *		
	65–74 years (n = 347)	75–84 (n = 214)	<0.001	2.34	1.62–3.36	0.006 *	1.97	1.21–3.20
		≥85 (n = 46)	<0.001	4.24	2.25–8.01	0.003 *	3.63	1.54–8.55
Gender	male (n = 246)	female (n = 361)	<0.001	2.30	1.60–3.30	0.211	0.65	0.34–1.26
Education						0.162		
	university-high (n = 54)	non-literate (n = 160)	<0.001	8.20	3.32–20.24	0.071	2.72	0.91–8.08
		quit prim. s. (n = 90)	0.001	5.09	1.97–13.14	0.082	2.69	0.88–8.20
		primary s. (n = 276)	0.011	3.15	1.29–7.66	0.259	1.80	0.64–5.00
		secondary s. (n = 27)	0.044	3.36	1.03–11.01	0.061	3.85	0.93–15.84
Marital status	married (n = 407)	widow (n = 200)	<0.001	2.95	2.07–4.21	0.494	1.65	0.39–7.04
Living						0.946		
	with spouse (n = 291)	living alone (n = 115)	<0.001	3.20	2.03–5.03	0.466	1.76	0.38–8.06
		spouse-child (n = 113)	0.359	1.25	0.77–2.03	0.584	1.18	0.64–2.15
		children (n = 75)	<0.001	3.29	1.94–5.57	0.582	1.52	0.33–6.92
		relative/carer (n = 13)	0.273	1.90	0.60–5.99	0.665	1.48	0.24–8.93
Economic						0.123		
	retired (n = 298)	no income (n = 140)	0.003	1.91	1.24–2.94	0.105	1.82	0.88–3.78
		aged wage (n = 53)	<0.001	3.51	1.92–6.41	0.544	1.29	0.56–2.95
		wage spouse (n = 116)	<0.001	2.83	1.80–4.44	0.397	0.72	0.35–1.51
Disability						0.027 *		
	no (n = 463)	blind (n = 42)	0.005	2.48	1.31–4.69	0.082	2.03	0.91–4.51
		hearing imp. (n = 57)	0.126	1.56	0.88–2.75	0.776	0.89	0.42–1.90
		walking imp. (n = 45)	<0.001	6.10	3.10–11.99	0.013 *	2.80	1.24–6.33
Fall history	no (n = 370)	yes (n = 237)	<0.001	3.39	2.39–4.81	<0.001 *	2.25	1.46–3.46
Number CD						0.205		
	no (n = 65)	1 (n = 117)	0.326	1.52	0.65–3.52	0.390	1.70	0.50–5.74
		2 (n = 160)	0.004	3.17	1.45–6.89	0.152	2.43	0.72–8.24
		3 (n = 109)	0.001	3.90	1.74–8.70	0.090	2.98	0.84–10.55
		≥4 (n = 156)	<0.001	6.55	3.03–14.15	0.047 *	3.54	1.01–12.32
Number MG						0.831		
	no (n = 78)	1 (n = 160)	0.265	1.47	0.74–2.91	0.450	0.65	0.22–1.95
		2 (n = 164)	0.011	2.37	1.22–4.59	0.524	0.70	0.23–2.09
		≥3 (n = 205)	<0.001	4.27	2.25–8.09	0.697	0.80	0.26–2.44
Incontinence						0.002 *		
	no (n = 343)	yes (n = 177)	<0.001	5.30	3.56–7.89	0.001 *	2.40	1.46–3.95
		sometimes (n = 87)	<0.001	2.75	1.66–4.54	0.057	1.81	0.98–3.35
Nocturia	no (n = 280)	yes (n = 327)	<0.001	2.83	1.98–4.05	0.577	1.14	0.71–1.81
Walking	yes (n = 384)	no (n = 223)	<0.001	4.18	2.93–5.97	0.001 *	2.21	1.41–3.48
LTA						0.079		
	3+ (n = 77)	no (n = 60)	<0.001	9.88	4.17–23.40	0.024 *	3.40	1.17–9.88
		1+2 (n = 470)	<0.001	4.08	1.98–8.40	0.097	2.04	0.87–4.77
BMI						0.093		
	<25 (n = 114)	25–29.9 (n = 217)	0.340	1.29	0.76–2.19	0.206	1.54	0.78–3.03
		30–34.9 (n = 170)	0.002	2.36	1.39–4.04	0.044 *	2.09	1.02–4.28
		≥35 (n = 106)	<0.001	3.25	1.82–5.82	0.019 *	2.53	1.16–5.50

* Statistically significant ($p < 0.05$), OR: Odds ratio, C.I.: Confidence interval, CD: Chronic disease, MG: Medication group, LTA: Leisure time activities, BMI: Body Mass Index, prim. s.: Primary school, s.: School, imp.: Impairment, ** Multiple logistic regression analysis with enter method.

The study included elderly participants who did not urinate while sleeping at night and those who got up and went to urinate two or more times at night. Nocturia was not statistically significantly associated with balance disorders.

A total of 63.2% of the participants (n = 384) stated that they went out of the house and walked to go to the market, street market, mosque, coffee shop, or park. A lack of walking was statistically significantly associated with balance disorders. Balance disorders were 2.21 times more prevalent in the participants who did not walk than in those who walked to the market or those who took walks in the park ($p = 0.001$, OR = 2.21, 95% CI = 1.41–3.48).

Participants were asked about hobbies and interests to learn about leisure time activities. Participants reported eight types of hobby activities. These activities included reading activities; artistic activities, such as painting, music, and poetry; sports activities, such as swimming, fishing, and hunting; gardening and field work; making handcrafts; using the computer, foundation memberships; and mental games like chess and puzzles. Participation in leisure time activities was not statistically significantly associated with balance disorders, but, compared with the elderly who participated in three or more leisure time activities, the prevalence of balance disorders in participants who did not participate in activities was 3.4 times higher ($p = 0.024$, OR = 3.4, 95% CI = 1.17–9.88).

The BMI values of participants were measured. Individuals were classified as normal weight (<25), overweight (25–29.9), obese (30–34.9), or overly obese (≥35). BMI was not statistically significantly associated with balance disorders, but, compared with the participants with BMI < 25, balance disorders were approximately two times more common in obese ($p = 0.044$, OR = 2.09, 95% CI = 1.02–4.28) and overly obese participants ($p = 0.019$, OR = 2.53, 95% CI = 1.16–5.50).

4. Discussion

In this study, the prevalence of balance disorders was found to be 34.3% in the community-dwelling elderly. Older age, physical disability, the presence of incontinence, having a history of falls, having four or more chronic illnesses, not walking regularly, absence of free time activity, and obesity were found to be associated with an increased prevalence of balance disorders.

International studies have investigated balance disorders in elderly individuals living in the community. In a study conducted in the UK in 2008, the prevalence of balance disorders was found to be 21.5% among elderly individuals living in the community [21]. In a study conducted in the United States that was published in 2012 including participants aged ≥65 years with an average age of 74.4 years, the prevalence of balance disorders was approximately 20% [22]. In a study conducted in Scotland published in 1994, the prevalence of balance disorders was found to be 30% [23]. In another BBS-based study published in the US in 2006 including 101 community-dwelling volunteers aged >65 years, the prevalence of balance disorders was found to be 32% [24]. In our study, we found the prevalence of balance disorders to be 34.3%, which is in good agreement with the literature.

Şahin and colleagues performed a Turkish validity and reliability study of the BBS in 2008 including 60 healthy individuals aged >65 years. The average BBS score in that study was 47.63 ± 9.88 [18]. In a study conducted by Soyuer et al. using the BBS, the average BBS score was 45.42 ± 12.11 in nursing home residents [25]. In another study, the average BBS score was 41.3 ± 9 [26]. We found an average score of 43.49 ± 14.23 in our study.

In a study about the effect of age on balance disorders, a decrease in BBS scores with age was reported [27]. In another study, increased age was associated with decreasing BBS scores [28]. In our study, we also found that balance disorders were significantly more common in those aged 75–84 years and in those aged >85 years than in those aged 65–74 years.

In a study published in 2012, in which the effect of gender on the prevalence of balance disorders was examined, the prevalence of balance disorders was reported to be higher in females than in males [22]. In another study published in 2013, BBS scores were lower for female participants [27]. However, gender was not found to be a meaningful variable in our study.

Regarding the relationship between visual disturbance, balance, and falls, visual disturbance was found to be associated with the prevalence of falling [29]. In another study, elderly patients with visual disorders were found to have lower balance scores than a control group [30]. In another study, peripheral visual loss was reported to have a negative effect on balance control [31]. In our study, although overall disability status was significantly associated with balance disorders, visual disability had no effect on balance. At the same time, walking impairment was associated with balance.

In a study published in 2012, one-third of participants with balance disorders participated in no exercise-related activities or social activities [22]. In our study, participants who did not walk and who did not participate in any free time activities had a high likelihood of having a balance disorder. Our data match those reported by others. In a study published in 2019, the effect of exercise on falls was reported. Sherrington et al. found that participation in exercise mainly involving balance

and functional exercises, plus resistance exercise, was associated with a reduction in falls. However, Sherrington et al. did not find enough evidence to determine the effect of walking programs on falls [32]. In contrast, in our study, we found a lower prevalence of balance disorders in those who walked regularly than in those who did not walk.

We think that the causes of balance disorders in elderly people with a walking disability and those who do not walk regularly may be sarcopenia and demineralization. It is known that the most important muscle for balance is the quadriceps femoris. We think that the loss of this muscle has a negative effect on balance in elderly people who do not walk regularly. In addition, loss of minerals from bone and decreased signal frequency from the proprioceptive receptors may have negative effects. As a result, we advise elderly people to walk regularly.

When we look at the relationship between postural balance and falls, posturographic vestibular rehabilitation has been reported to improve balance in elderly individuals and to reduce the number of falls [33]. Impaired balance has been reported as one of the long term risk factors for falls in men [34]. In another study, participants were classified into the non-fall group, one-time fall group, and repeated fall group. Both the dynamic balance and static balance scores were found to be higher in the non-fall group than in the one-time fall group and repeated fall group [35]. In our study, the prevalence of balance disorders was found to be significantly higher in people with a fall history.

In a study that was conducted to show the relationship between balance disorders and a fear of falling, the presence of balance, gait, and cognitive disorders was reported to be significantly higher in elderly individuals with a fear of falling [36]. In another study that used the Berg Balance Scale, lower BBS scores were found in the group with a fear of falling compared to those in the group without a fear of falling [27]. In our study, the presence of balance disorders was found to be significantly higher in those who had a fear of falling than in those who did not have a fear of falling ($p < 0.001$) (Table 1).

In a study on obesity in the elderly, an increased Body Mass Index (BMI) was associated with decreases in both dynamic stability and balance in the elderly [37]. In a study published in 2018, older participants were classified into obese, normal weight, and weak groups according to Body Mass Index scores. The one-leg standing time test was applied to determine balance scores. In the obese group, the one-leg standing time was much shorter than in the normal weight group of community-dwelling elderly women [38]. In our study, the prevalence of balance disorders was found to be higher in obese (BMI = 30–34.9) and overly obese (BMI ≥ 35) elderly individuals ($p = 0.044$ and $p = 0.019$, respectively) than in individuals of normal weight.

Balance disorders, incontinence, fall history, and age have been associated with each other in many studies published in this area [39,40]. These variables were found to be significant in the multiple logistic regression analysis in our study, too.

Our study had both limitations and significant contributions. In terms of limitations, some of the survey data were determined from the statements of elderly individuals—fall history, for example. In addition, the participants in our study consisted of elderly people living in a district center, and different socio-demographic data could be obtained from elderly people living in other parts of the country. In terms of contributions, to our knowledge, no previous study in this area has been conducted in Turkey using the stratified random sampling method to interview a large sample of community-dwelling elderly individuals face-to-face at their homes. We were able to get the right data because we applied the BBS test. In addition to academic data, our study also guided a local government social project. Walking support materials (walking stick, walker, wheelchair) were given to the elderly who were identified as having a balance disorder. Our work has created awareness in the community (see Appendix A).

Our research data may be used as reference for other academic studies in this area. The identification of the relationship between equilibrium and falling in the elderly and the emergence of many health and social causes of balance disorders are very valuable. More work is needed to determine the mechanisms behind each of these reasons. Awareness of these causes is needed for both individual and social preventive health practices. Following the collection of these data, people have learned that they need to change their lifestyles to protect their health. The local government has launched projects to support elderly people after obtaining these data. It has opened courses where seniors can spend their leisure time, with picture, music, craft, and folklore courses. Using the sociodemographic data of the elderly collected in this study, a journal called "Old Age Atlas of Söke" was published in the district. Söke Municipality published this journal to district people. This journal increased the awareness of people in the district about old age and old age problems. The social contributions of the study were appreciated by people in the district in addition to the academic contributions.

Balance disorders, which are considered to have several biological and social etiologies, are a major geriatric problem which lead leading to falling and increased morbidity and mortality rates. The development of national health and social policies that address the underlying causes of this problem and the introduction of preventive health care services should be the primary steps towards helping today's increasingly elderly population. The concept of "age-friendly" should be widespread in all segments of the society, including the private sector and public services.

Author Contributions: Conceptualization, T.B.D., S.F.A., and E.S.S.; methodology, T.B.D. and S.F.A.; validation, T.B.D.; investigation, T.B.D.; writing—original draft preparation, T.B.D.; writing—review and editing, T.B.D., Z.F.S., and E.S.S.; supervision, T.B.D. and Z.F.S.; project administration, Z.F.S. and S.F.A.; funding acquisition, Z.F.S. and E.S.S.

Funding: This research was funded by Ege University Medical Faculty Scientific Research Projects Commission (protocol number 2016 TIP–031).

Acknowledgments: This manuscript was prepared as part of the PhD thesis of the corresponding author. It was also partially summarized at the International Academic Geriatrics Congress 2017 as an oral presentation. We would like to thank Timur KÖSE and retired Oktay TEKEŞİN for their support with this study.

Conflicts of Interest: The authors declare no conflict of interest. The funders had no role in the design of the study; in the collection, analyses, or interpretation of data; in the writing of the manuscript, or in the decision to publish the results.

Appendix A.

In addition to the academic content of our study, a social aspect was also included. Walking support materials (walking stick, walker, wheelchair) were given to the elderly people who were identified as having a balance disorder. These support materials were gifted to the elderly by Söke Municipality to allow them to participate in a social life and to protect them from falls. The data from our study allowed us to implement a project called "age-friendly municipality."

References

1. Sturnieks, D.L.; St George, R.; Lord, S.R. Balance disorders in the elderly. *Neurophysiol. Clin.* **2008**, *38*, 467–478. [CrossRef] [PubMed]
2. Nnodim, J.O.; Yung, R.L. Balance and its clinical assessment in older adults—A review. *J. Geriatr. Med. Gerontol.* **2015**, *1*, 003. [CrossRef]
3. Perera, T.; Tan, J.L.; Cole, M.H.; Yohanandan, S.A.C.; Silberstein, P.; Cook, R.; Peppard, R.; Aziz, T.; Coyne, T.; Brown, P.; et al. Balance control systems in Parkinson's disease and the impact of pedunculopontine area stimulation. *Brain* **2018**, *141*, 3009–3022. [CrossRef]
4. Cameron, I.D.; Dyer, S.M.; Panagoda, C.E.; Murray, G.R.; Hill, K.D.; Cumming, R.G.; Kerse, N. Interventions for preventing falls in older people in care facilities and hospitals. *Cochrane Database Syst. Rev.* **2018**, 9. [CrossRef]
5. Bergen, G.; Stevens, M.R.; Burns, E.R. Falls and fall injuries among adults aged ≥65 years—United States, 2014. *MMWR Morb. Mortal. Wkly. Rep.* **2016**, *65*, 993–998. [CrossRef]
6. Covington, D.L.; Maxwell, J.G.; Clancy, T.V. Hospital resources used to treat the injured elderly at North Carolina trauma centers. *J. Am. Geriatr. Soc.* **1993**, *41*, 847–852. [CrossRef]
7. Onat, Ş.Ş.; Delialioğlu, S.Ü.; Özel, S. The relationship of balance between functional status and quality of life in the geriatric population. *Turk. J. Phys. Med. Rehabil.* **2014**, *60*, 147–154. [CrossRef]

8. Nguyen, T.Q.; Young, J.H.; Rodriguez, A.; Zupancic, S.; Lie, D.Y.C. Differentiation of patients with balance insufficiency (vestibular hypofunction) versus normal subjects using a low-cost small wireless wearable gait sensor. *Biosensors* **2019**, *9*, 29. [CrossRef] [PubMed]
9. Von Brevern, M.; Radtke, A.; Lezius, F.; Feldmann, M.; Ziese, T.; Lempert, T.; Neuhauser, H. Epidemiology of benign paroxysmal positional vertigo: A population based study. *J. Neurol Neurosurg. Psychiatr.* **2007**, *78*, 710–715. [CrossRef] [PubMed]
10. Felsenthal, G.; Ference, T.S.; Young, M.A. Aging of organ systems. In *Downey and Darling's Physiological Basis of Rehabilitation Medicine*, 3th ed.; Gonzales, E.G., Myers, S.A., Edelstein, J.E., Lieberman, J.S., Downey, J.A., Eds.; Butterwoth Heinemann: Boston, MA, USA, 2001; pp. 561–577.
11. Salzman, B. Gait and balance disorders in older adults. *Am. Fam. Physician* **2010**, *82*, 61–68.
12. World Health Organization. WHO global report on falls prevention in older age. 2007, pp. 15–18. Available online: https://www.who.int/ageing/publications/Falls_prevention7March.pdf (accessed on 23 February 2019).
13. Turkey Healthy Aging Action Plan and Implementation Programme 2015–2020, Ankara. 2015; p. 33. Available online: https://sbu.saglik.gov.tr/Ekutuphane/kitaplar/Sağl\T1\ikl\T1\i%20Yaş.%202015--2020%20Pdf.pdf (accessed on 24 February 2019). (In Turkish)
14. Güngen, C.; Ertan, T.; Eker, E.; Yaşar, R.; Engin, F. Reliability and Validity of The Standardized Mini Mental State Examination in The Diagnosis of Mild Dementia in Turkish Population. *Turk. J. Psychiatry* **2002**, *13*, 273–281.
15. Berg, K.O.; Maki, B.E.; Williams, J.I.; Holliday, P.J.; Wood-Dauphinee, S.L. Clinical and laboratory measures of postural balance in an elderly population. *Arch. Phys. Med. Rehabil.* **1992**, *73*, 1073–1080.
16. Berg, K.; Wood-Dauphinee, S.; Williams, J.I.; Maki, B. Measuring balance in the elderly: Validation of an instrument. *Can. J. Pub. Health* **1992**, *2*, 7–11.
17. Berg, K.; Wood-Dauphinee, S.; Williams, J.I. The Balance Scale: Reliability assessment with elderly residents and patients with an acute stroke. *Scand. J. Rehabil. Med.* **1995**, *27*, 27–36. [PubMed]
18. Sahin, F.; Yilmaz, F.; Ozmaden, A.; Kotevolu, N.; Sahin, T.; Kuran, B. Reliability and validity of the Turkish version of the Berg Balance Scale. *J. Geriatr. Phys. Ther.* **2008**, *31*, 32–37. [CrossRef]
19. Kornetti, D.L.; Fritz, S.L.; Chiu, Y.P.; Light, K.E.; Velozo, C.A. Rating scale analysis of the Berg Balance Scale. *Arch. Phys. Med. Rehabil.* **2004**, *85*, 1128–1135. [CrossRef] [PubMed]
20. Dogan, A.; Mengulluoglu, M.; Ozgırgın, N. Evaluation of the effect of ankle-foot orthosis use on balance and mobility in hemiparetic stroke patients. *Disabil. Rehabil.* **2011**, *33*, 1433–1439. [CrossRef]
21. Stevens, K.N.; Lang, I.A.; Guralnik, J.M.; Melzer, D. Epidemiology of balance and dizziness in a national population: Findings from the English Longitudinal Study of Ageing. *Age Ageing* **2008**, *37*, 300–305. [CrossRef]
22. Lin, H.W.; Bhattacharyya, N. Balance Disorders in the elderly: Epidemiology and functional impact. *Laryngoscope* **2012**, *122*, 1858–1861. [CrossRef]
23. Colledge, N.R.; Wilson, J.A.; Macintyre, C.C.; Mac Lennan, W.J. The prevalence and characteristics of dizziness in an elderly community. *Age Ageing* **1994**, *23*, 117–120. [CrossRef]
24. Hawk, C.; Hyland, J.K.; Rupert, R.; Colonvega, M.; Hall, S. Assessment of balance and risk for falls in a sample of community-dwelling adults aged 65 and older. *Chiropr. Osteopat.* **2006**, *14*, 3. [CrossRef]
25. Soyuer, F.; Şenol, V.; Elmalı, F. Physical activity, balance and mobility functions of individuals over 65 years of age in the nursing homes. *Van Med. J.* **2012**, *19*, 116–121. (In Turkish). Available online: https://www.journalagent.com/vtd/pdfs/VTD_19_3_116_121.pdf. (accessed on 5 February 2019).
26. Holbein-Jenny, M.A.; Billek-Sawhney, B.; Beckman, E.; Smith, T. Balance in personal care home residents: A comparison of the Berg Balance Scale, the Multi-Directional Reach Test, and the Activities-Specific Balance Confidence Scale. *J. Geriatr. Phys. Ther.* **2005**, *28*, 48–53. [CrossRef]
27. Ulus, Y.; Akyol, Y.; Tander, B.; Durmuş, D.; Bilgici, A.; Kuru, Ö. The relationship between fear of falling and balance in community-dwelling older people. *Turk. J. Geriatr.* **2013**, *16*, 260–265. Available online: http://geriatri.dergisi.org/uploads/pdf/pdf_TJG_745.pdf. (accessed on 11 February 2019).
28. Steffen, T.M.; Hacker, T.A.; Mollinger, L. Age and gender related test performance in community-dwelling elderly people: Six-minute walk test, Berg Balance Scale, timed up-go test and gait speeds. *Physical. Ther.* **2002**, *82*, 128–137. [CrossRef]

29. Guimarães, J.M.N.; Farinatti, P.T.V. Descriptive analysis of variables theoretically associated to the risk of falls in elder women. *Rev. Bras. Med. Esport.* **2005**, *11*, 280–286. Available online: http://www.scielo.br/pdf/rbme/v11n5/en_27593.pdf. (accessed on 11 February 2019).
30. Popescu, M.L.; Boisjoly, H.; Schmaltz, H.; Kergoat, M.J.; Rousseau, J.; Moghadaszadeh, S.; Djafari, F.; Freeman, E.E. Age-related eye disease and mobility limitations in older adults. *Invest. Ophthalmol. Vis. Sci.* **2011**, *9*, 7168–7174. [CrossRef]
31. Kotecha, A.; Chopra, R.; Fahy, R.T.; Rubin, G.S. Dual tasking and balance in those with central and peripheral vision loss. *Invest. Ophthalmol Vis. Sci.* **2013**, *54*, 5408–5415. [CrossRef] [PubMed]
32. Sherrington, C.; Fairhall, N.J.; Wallbank, G.K.; Tiedemann, A.; Michaleff, Z.A.; Howard, K.; Clemson, L.; Hopewell, S.; Lamb, S.E. Exercise for preventing falls in older people living in the community. *Cochrane Database Syst. Rev.* **2019**, *31*. [CrossRef]
33. Soto-Varela, A.; Gayoso-Diz, P.; Faraldo-García, A.; Rossi-Izquierdo, M.; Vaamonde-Sánchez-Andrade, I.; Del-Río-Valeiras, M.; Lirola-Delgado, A.; Santos-Pérez, S. Optimising costs in reducing rate of falls in older people with the improvement of balance by means of vestibular rehabilitation (ReFOVeRe study): A randomized controlled trial comparing computerised dynamic posturography vs. mobile vibrotactile posturography system. *BMC Geriatr.* **2019**, *19*, 1. [CrossRef]
34. Ek, S.; Rizzuto, D.; Fratiglioni, L.; Calderón-Larrañaga, A.; Johnell, K.; Sjöberg, L.; Xu, W.; Welmer, A.K. Risk factors for injurious falls in older adults: The role of sex and length of follow-up. *J. Am. Geriatr Soc.* **2019**, *67*, 246–253. [CrossRef]
35. Jeon, M.; Gu, M.O.; Yim, J. Comparison of Walking, Muscle Strength, Balance, and Fear of Falling Between Repeated Fall Group, One-time Fall Group, and Nonfall Group of the ElderlyReceiving Home Care Service. *Asian Nurs. Res. (Korean Soc. Nurs. Sci).* **2017**, *11*, 290–296. [CrossRef]
36. Vellas, B.J.; Wayne, S.J.; Romero, L.J.; Baumgartner, R.N.; Garry, P.J. Fear of falling and restriction of mobility in elderly fallers. *Age Ageing* **1997**, *26*, 189–193. [CrossRef]
37. Gao, X.; Wang, L.; Shen, F.; Ma, Y.; Fan, Y.; Niu, H. Dynamic walking stability of elderly people with various BMIs. *Gait Posture* **2019**, *68*, 168–173. [CrossRef]
38. Nonaka, K.; Murata, S.; Shiraiwa, K.; Abiko, T.; Nakano, H.; Iwase, H.; Naito, K.; Horie, J. Physical characteristics vary according to body mass index in Japanese community-dwelling elderly women. *Geriatrics* **2018**, *3*, 87. [CrossRef]
39. Tkacheva, O.N.; Runikhina, N.K.; Ostapenko, V.S.; Sharashkina, N.V.; Mkhitaryan, E.A.; Onuchina, J.S.; Lysenkov, S.N.; Yakhno, N.N.; Press, Y. Prevalence of geriatric syndromes among people aged 65 years and older at four community clinics in Moscow. *Clin. Interv. Aging.* **2018**, *13*, 251–259. [CrossRef]
40. Almeida Abreu, H.C.; Oliveira Reiners, A.A.; Souza Azevedo, R.C.; Silva, A.M.C.; Oliveira Moura Abreu, D.R.; Oliveira, A.D. Incidence and predicting factors of falls of older inpatients. *Rev. Saude Publica* **2015**, *49*. [CrossRef]

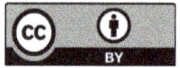

© 2019 by the authors. Licensee MDPI, Basel, Switzerland. This article is an open access article distributed under the terms and conditions of the Creative Commons Attribution (CC BY) license (http://creativecommons.org/licenses/by/4.0/).

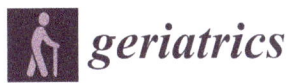

Review

Geriatric Assessment in Multicultural Immigrant Populations

Katherine T. Ward [1,2,*], Mailee Hess [1,2] and Shirley Wu [1,2]

1. Section of Geriatrics, Division of General Internal Medicine, Department of Medicine, Harbor-UCLA Medical Center, Torrance, CA 90509, USA
2. David Geffen School of Medicine at UCLA, Los Angeles, CA 90095, USA
* Correspondence: kward@dhs.lacounty.gov

Received: 16 May 2019; Accepted: 20 June 2019; Published: 26 June 2019

Abstract: While the traditional comprehensive geriatric assessment provides valuable information essential to caring for older adults, it often falls short in multicultural immigrant populations. The number of foreign-born older adults is growing, and in some regions of the United States of America (U.S.), they encompass a significant portion of the older adult population. To ensure we are caring for this culturally diverse population adequately, we need to develop a more culturally competent comprehensive geriatric assessment. In this review, we explore ways in which to do this, address areas unique to multicultural immigrant populations, and identify limitations of the current assessment tools when applied to these populations. In order to be more culturally sensitive, we should incorporate the concepts of ethnogeriatrics into a comprehensive geriatric assessment, by addressing topics like healthcare disparities, language barriers, health literacy, acculturation level, and culturally defined beliefs. Additionally, we must be sensitive to the limitations of our current assessment tools and consider how we can expand our assessment toolkit to address these limitations. We discuss the limitations in cognitive screening tests, delirium assessments, functional and mental health assessments, advance care planning, and elder abuse.

Keywords: multicultural; geriatric assessment; ethnogeriatrics; immigrant; social determinants

1. Introduction: Geriatric Assessment in Multicultural Immigrant Populations

The comprehensive geriatric assessment has proven to be a valuable tool to address the health and wellness of the older adult population. However, geriatric assessment tools were developed within Western biomedical models that may not apply to all subpopulations of older adults in the United States of America (U.S.). In this paper, we seek to review and recommend best practices on approaching geriatric assessment in a multicultural immigrant population. We explore the challenges that need to be considered for the geriatric assessment in a multicultural immigrant population, the evidence that highlights the inadequacy of our current assessment, and some potential solutions to improve our geriatric assessments.

In 2001, the Institute of Medicine published "Retooling for an Aging America," describing the need for a health care workforce that can address the diversity of the aging population in the U.S. and suggesting that the health of individuals depends on more than just their vital signs, laboratory tests, or physical examinations; individual health is influenced by culture, language, national origin, religion, education, income and assets, level of acculturation, and more [1]. Addressing these issues requires that policy-makers and health care providers be familiar with the individual patient's health beliefs, risk for diseases, family systems, access to care, and dependency on adult children.

The U.S. population encompasses approximately 50 million immigrants, and census data suggest that 15% of adults 60 years and older are foreign-born [2]. This population is expected to increase; the proportion of foreign-born older adults in 2030 is estimated to be 25%, increasing to 35% by 2050 [3].

The foreign-born population is not geographically uniform. In California, foreign-born older adults comprise more than a third of the older adult population; in Los Angeles County, this population approaches 50%. A more culturally sensitive approach to geriatrics is particularly important in these communities.

Undocumented older adult immigrants have additional needs, and this population is expected to grow rapidly over the next 15 years. Eleven million immigrants in the U.S. are undocumented, of which 10% are currently older than 55. Undocumented older adult immigrants face additional challenges beyond serious chronic health issues, including cognitive disorders and physical injuries with functional impairment. They may work and pay into Social Security and Medicare, yet are unable to claim these benefits as they age due to their undocumented status. They often have poor access to health care and do not receive primary preventive care, which results in more expensive care [3]. Furthermore, they are also at increased risk for elder abuse; their immigration status and fear of deportation is a vulnerability that can be exploited [4,5].

2. Challenges to the Geriatric Evaluation in a Multicultural Immigrant Population

While cross-cultural health care has been taught in health professions training programs since the 1970s, it was not until the 1990s that it was adapted to geriatric training programs. Around that time, the term "ethnogeriatrics" emerged and was defined as culturally competent health care for older adults [6]. A curricular framework for multicultural geriatric care was created and intended to be adaptable to various academic programs. The curriculum includes, for example, the effects of health care disparities, language, health literacy, acculturation level, and culturally defined beliefs [7]. Each of these aspects can have effects on the patient's health directly but can also affect the provider's assessment in areas of cognition, mood, and function. The topics of ethnogeriatrics are not typically included in the traditional comprehensive geriatric assessment, and yet are necessary to adequately care for immigrant older adult populations.

In addition, we also need better assessment instruments. The traditional comprehensive geriatric assessment tools have infrequently been validated in a multicultural immigrant geriatric population and, therefore, limit the provider's ability to achieve high-quality multicultural care. For instance, cognitive tests are not validated for all languages, and most are not validated for populations with no formal education [8–10]. If an assessment tool has been studied in one ethnic group, it may not be applicable to a multicultural immigrant population as a whole.

In Table 1, we summarize an approach to geriatric immigrant multicultural assessment and identify gaps that are opportunities for improvement. Gaps range widely depending on the existing literature. Several elements require the development of new assessment tools, others have existing tools that may need further validation in immigrant populations, and some need further downstream development and validation of interventions that improve outcomes in these populations.

2.1. Health Care Disparities

Health care disparities are differences in health and health care among population groups. Health disparities and delayed health care among older adults have been found to be negatively associated with both self-reported health and mental health status. For example, population studies have found that foreign-born Asians and Latinos have the poorest self-reported health and mental health [11].

Due to the dramatic disparities in a multicultural immigrant population, the geriatric assessment should include an evaluation of which health conditions were delayed in diagnosis and treatment. For example, newly diagnosed diabetes needs to be treated, as well as the sequelae of delayed diagnosis, such as visual loss from diabetic retinopathy or diabetic kidney disease.

Table 1. Elements of a Multicultural Geriatric Assessment.

Multicultural Assessment	Domain	Suggested Assessment Tools or Approach	Future Directions
1.	Baseline Preventive Care	Determine prior access to medical care, vaccination status, cancer screening history	Develop consensus guidelines on approach to vaccination assessment, cancer screening in older adult immigrant populations
2.	Chronic Conditions	Determine if diagnosis was delayed and address sequelae of untreated illness	
3.	Language	Determine literacy level and preferred language	
4.	Communication Barriers	Screen for cognitive, hearing, and visual impairment	Develop hearing loss screening assessment that can be used with an interpreter
5.	Health Literacy	Determine education level, print literacy, use teach-back method	Enhance low-literacy patient education in multiple languages. Develop and validate training for Community Health Workers (CHWs) on health coaching in older adult immigrant populations.
6.	Acculturation Level	Assess self-reported health	Conduct longitudinal studies of self-reported health in older adult immigrants and correlate with health outcomes

Traditional Geriatric Assessment	Domain	Suggested Assessment Tools or Approach	Future Directions
1.	Cognitive	Rowland Universal Dementia Assessment Scale (RUDAS)	Validate RUDAS in more subpopulations. Develop new low-literacy cognitive screening tools.
2.	Delirium	Vigilance testing (e.g., A test), CAM-ICU in preferred language	Develop delirium screening tools for use with interpreters.
3.	Mental Health	Geriatric Depression Scale (GDS)	Modify existing tools or develop new culturally specific depression screening tools. Further evaluate outcomes with treatment of depression.
4.	Functional Evaluation	Assess the application of change in basic and instrumental activities of daily living, determine cultural expectations for Activities of Daily Living (ADLs) for older adults	Modify existing functional assessment tools to be culturally specific.
5.	Advance Care Planning and Decision-Making	Determine culturally defined beliefs regarding health and symptomatology, information sharing, and preferred decision-maker	Further studies are needed on advance care planning in older adult immigrant populations.
6.	Elder Abuse and Mistreatment	Determine immigration status (or ask if patient is willing to share documentation status)	Develop culturally sensitive and brief screening tools

Completion of preventive health care, such as vaccinations and cancer screening, is low in the immigrant older adult population [12]. Evidence-based guidelines do not address how to approach cancer screening in older adults who have passed the age of screening but who have not completed prior screenings. For example, do you screen for breast cancer in a 70-year-old woman with no prior breast cancer screenings?

2.2. Language

The geriatric assessment should include identifying the preferred language of the patient and strategies for addressing communication barriers.

Language barriers are an added complexity for a medical visit in any age group. While medical interpreters or telephone-based interpreter services are frequently utilized and mandated by The National Enhanced Culturally and Linguistically Appropriate Services Standards (CLAS) [13,14], using interpreters to communicate is time-consuming and an added challenge in a busy medical setting.

Older adults have additional issues that can make communicating through interpreter services even more challenging, especially when using phone or video interpreters. Cognitive impairment and hearing impairment are frequently encountered in older adult populations and require additional time and patience [15]. If patients cannot hear the phone interpreter because of hearing impairment or do not understand how to use the interpreter because of cognitive impairment, family members are often relied upon to help with communicating with the patient. Although there may not be good alternatives, it is important to understand that this comes with risks. If family members do not speak English, a message will be repeated multiple times with a provider speaking to the interpreter who then speaks to the family member who then speaks to the patient. Alternatively, when family members do speak English, they often do not interpret directly but try to answer for the patient, resulting in the patient being removed from the conversation completely. Additionally, when family members are used to interpret, patients may refrain from discussing details or topics they do not want family members to know or to worry about. Although it has not been well studied, there is evidence that language barriers have some effect on patient safety and certainly can play a role in the provider's ability to elicit patient symptoms, resulting in diagnostic errors [16].

Repetition using the "teach-back" method may improve information transfer [17]. When obtaining a history from a patient who does not speak the same language, summary statements and repeating back can help ensure accurate history-taking. Most interventions improving information transfer recommend the "teach-back" technique to ensure understanding.

2.3. Health Literacy

Print literacy is the ability to read or write; health literacy is the degree to which individuals can understand, communicate, and act upon health information. Low health literacy can affect patients' ability to follow through on a treatment plan, take medications correctly, or even understand what medical problems they have. Older adults, immigrants, minorities, and individuals with low incomes are more likely to have low health literacy. However, the inability to read and write or having a low educational level also contributes to low health literacy. The lack of understanding health information can theoretically lead to difficulty in engaging in health behaviors, preventative services, and disease management [18]. Health outcomes that have been measured related to low health literacy showed an increase in all-cause mortality rate [19] and a continual decline in baseline physical functioning [20].

While screening tools for health literacy exist, they are often impractical for the clinic setting. The concern for low health literacy is typically uncovered when working with patients directly. For instance, when discussing what they understand about their medical conditions or even obtaining a detailed history on whether they know when and which medicine to take can be enlightening. Documenting the concern for low health literacy can be helpful to communicate with other providers or specialists caring for the patient, but even more importantly, documenting possible solutions for addressing low health literacy can assist other providers to more effectively care for the patient [21].

Unstudied approaches to address health literacy include embedding community health workers (C.H.W.) in the team caring for the patient, or bringing the patient back for frequent nurse visits to manage chronic medical conditions such as hypertension and diabetes. When giving instructions about a treatment plan like how to take a medication, using teach-back methods can be helpful in ensuring patients understand what is being communicated. Additionally, involving other family members provides another layer of support.

2.4. Acculturation Level

Acculturation is the dynamic process that commences when an immigrant enters into a new country and begins to adapt to its culture. The long-term consequences of the acculturation process are highly variable, difficult to study, and depend on social and personal variables of the society of origin and the society of settlement [22]. Studies have used different measures of acculturation, including language proficiency, leading to inconsistencies in the relationship between acculturation and health outcomes [23]. Self-reported health has a predictive role in clinical outcomes and mortality and is thought to be a reliable measure for monitoring population health [24]. One systematic review of nine studies showed an association between acculturation and fair to poor self-related health in non-white immigrants compared to Caucasians [25]. Longitudinal studies are needed that focus on measurements of self-related health at the time of immigration and across several years of the acculturation process.

2.5. Culturally Defined Beliefs

Three important culturally influenced beliefs should be assessed: (1) patients' preferences for hearing health information and engaging in decision-making, (2) patients' cultural perception of illness, and (3) the role of spirituality and religion in patients' health [26]. Before these assessments, it is important to identify and respect older adults' preferences for hearing health information and making their own health care decisions. For instance, do patients want to hear about illness directly from the provider or do they prefer that information is given to family first, who then decide what the patient should know? If the patients do not want to hear information about their illness, then they should not be their own primary healthcare decision-makers. There needs to be at least one person who can weigh the risks and benefits of treatments and diagnostic procedures and can therefore provide informed consent. Determining the appropriate decision-maker and respecting patients' preferred communication parameters may help avoid communication breakdowns between providers and families.

Patients' perceptions of their illness and how they view the presentation of their illness is worth noting [27,28]. Using patients' terminology and symptomatology can help bridge communication barriers. Additionally, understanding the importance of spirituality and religion for patients and how this shapes their view of their health can also be helpful. Spiritual advisors or native healers in the healthcare team should be included as appropriate [29,30].

3. Elements of the Geriatric Assessment

Validated tools in the typical assessment have limitations: they often do not account for cultural differences, language barriers, health literacy, or education level. Using these tools can lead to misdiagnosis of geriatric syndromes and missed opportunities to help older adults. While all areas of the geriatric assessment may benefit from a more culturally sensitive approach, in this section, we address the six main areas for which the most literature exists: cognitive impairment, delirium, mental health, function, advance care planning, and elder abuse.

3.1. Cognitive Evaluation

The number of immigrants with dementia is expected to rise [31]. Unfortunately, our commonly used tools for diagnosing dementia are problematic in populations with low English proficiency and low literacy. Brief cognitive tests are necessary to screen for or confirm a suspected dementia, yet many of the tests currently used have been shown to underestimate cognitive abilities in patients with low English proficiency and low literacy. This leads to an underestimation of the cognitive abilities of the patient and an overdiagnosis of cognitive impairment or dementia [8]. Other evidence suggests that using an interpreter for cognitive testing may significantly affect the scores for neuropsychological testing, further complicating the evaluation [32]. In a review of multiple different cognitive tests for suspected dementia, investigators found that the Rowland Universal Dementia Assessment Scale (RUDAS) performed the best in a low-English proficiency and low-literacy population. Furthermore, when compared to the Mini Mental Status Exam, the RUDAS had more diagnostic accuracy in a memory clinic population with very low education [33]. Until better information or validated tools specifically addressing this population become available, we recommend using the RUDAS for screening in populations with low education levels and with low English proficiency.

3.2. Delirium Evaluation

Additional care must be given for attention testing when evaluating for delirium. While tests like reciting the months of the year backwards or the days of the week backwards are reasonable attention tests in English [34], this is not true for all languages. In many languages, days of the week and months of the year are numbers instead of separate and distinct words. For example, in Chinese, the days of the week backwards would be 6, 5, 4, and so on; therefore, reciting them backwards is a fundamentally different task from reciting day names backwards, such as Sunday, Saturday, Friday, and so on. For languages that do not have distinct words for months or days, using a vigilance test, such as identifying letters or characters in a series, may be more appropriate. In the A vigilance test, the patient is instructed to squeeze the provider's hand when they hear the letter A, then the provider spells out the phrase "S-A-V-E-A-H-A-A-R-T". While the Confusion Assessment Method for the Intensive Care Unit (CAM-ICU) has been translated and validated in multiple languages which can be found on the Vanderbilt Critical Illness, Brain Dysfunction and Survivorship Center website, most of these tools are written and validated for a provider who reads and speaks the patient's primary language and not necessarily for use with an interpreter [35].

3.3. Mental Health Evaluation

There are known disparities in adequate provider recognition of mental health issues due to language differences, health literacy barriers, and culturally specific presentations of distress. Furthermore, trained interpreters—even medical interpreters—may not be able to identify and interpret mental health issues during a geriatric evaluation. The level of acculturation and culturally defined beliefs can influence the mental health evaluation of a geriatric assessment [36].

There is a known gap in the literature about primary care-based depression screening for patients with limited English proficiency, best documented in the Spanish-speaking population. None of the used tests were found to be superior, however, fair evidence showed that the Geriatric Depression Scale (GDS) performed best in this population [37,38]. In addition to screening for depression, there is limited research on depression in older adult immigrants. Out of 80,000 studies looking at depression in the immigrant population, only 19 included older adults. Most of these studies did not mention cultural adaptations and its relationship to the presentation of depression. None of the studies examined the role of cultural background and patients' experience of anxiety or depression. In a collaborative care program of geriatric Latino immigrants, patients used a variety of idioms to describe their experiences with depression, potentially making screening more difficult in this population; bilingual psychotherapists provided the best environment to express patients' emotions and find solutions to problems [39]. While this may be the best solution in a multicultural immigrant population, this is not always available.

3.4. Functional Evaluation

Culturally based functional assessments methods assume familiarity with Western-centric culture. There is a tendency to overclassify impairments in immigrants. Also, not addressed in the Western-centric functional status evaluation are the unique gender and family roles that each culture brings to the functional evaluation [40]. For example, often times, adult children who sponsor their immigrant parents take over instrumental activities of daily living such as financial management, transportation, and shopping. Clinicians inadvertently judge this as a functional impairment. While there are more detailed ways to evaluate function such as the Clinical Dementia Rating [41], they take much longer to administer and are not practical in a clinical setting. Specific scales of function exist for many different cultures, for example, the Everyday Abilities Scale for India [42]. However, it is not practical for providers to know what individual assessment is appropriate for each culture they may be caring for, and this also makes functional assessments less generalizable and difficult to study.

3.5. Advance Care Planning and Decision-Making

Other important evaluations in the geriatric comprehensive assessment, which requires a more unique approach in a multicultural immigrant population, include beliefs on the use of advance directives, health care decision-making, disclosure and consent, gender issues, and issues related to the end of life [43]. Some cultures favor family- and community-centered health care decision-making over autonomy. Some people believe that bad news hastens death and therefore prefer very little information over truth telling. Some cultures value struggle at the end of life over comfort. This is an area that would benefit from further research.

3.6. Elder Abuse

Elder abuse and self-neglect are particularly troubling problems for older adults. National studies report a prevalence of 1 in 10 older adults experiencing abuse [44]. These numbers are even higher among minority populations, with one study in a Latino Spanish-speaking community of Los Angeles reporting a prevalence of elder abuse as high as 40% [4]. The use of Spanish-speaking "promotores" in this study, who were surveyors from the community and spoke the language of the study participants, was one of the hypothesized explanations for such high reported rates of elder abuse. The participants may have felt more comfortable disclosing sensitive information to someone whom they felt understood their own culture. This underscores how crucial it is for providers to be culturally sensitive if we are to have any chance at identifying abuse in these populations. Additionally, it is important to recognize that for undocumented immigrant populations, the fear of retaliation or deportation is a barrier for patients to report abuse.

4. Conclusions

In summary, there is a growing need for a more culturally sensitive comprehensive geriatric assessment in order to adequately address the complex social and cultural needs of immigrant older adults. Multicultural geriatric immigrant populations have unique circumstances that can have significant effects on their overall health and wellbeing and are typically not assessed with the traditional comprehensive geriatric assessment. Table 1 summarizes a rubric for best practices in a geriatric immigrant multicultural assessment and identifies gaps in the existing approaches. There is a need for further research and development of assessment tools that can be applied to a multicultural population.

Author Contributions: Conceptualization, K.T.W.; content, K.T.W. and M.H.; writing—original draft preparation, K.T.W.; writing—review and editing, K.T.W., M.H., and S.W.

Funding: This research received no external funding

Conflicts of Interest: The authors declare no conflict of interest.

References

1. Institute of Medicine (US) Committee on the Future Health Care Workforce for Older Americans. *Retooling for an Aging America: Building the Health Care Workforce*; The National Academies Press: Washington, DC, USA, 2008.
2. U.S. Census. *2015 Summary Files 1,2,3, & 4*; 2016. Available online: https://census.gov (accessed on 11 May 2019).
3. Wiltz, T. Aging, Undocumented and Uninsured Immigrants Challenge Cites and States. Stateline Article 2018. Available online: https://www.pewtrusts.org/en/research-and-analysis/blogs/stateline/2018/01/03/aging-undocumented-and-uninsured-immigrants-challenge-cities-and-states. (accessed on 11 May 2019).
4. DeLiema, M.; Gassoumis, Z.D.; Homeier, D.C.; Wilber, K.H. Determining prevalence and correlates of elder abuse using promotores: Low-income immigrant latinos report high rates of abuse and neglect. *J. Am. Geriat. Soc.* **2012**, *60*, 1333–1339. [CrossRef] [PubMed]
5. Montoya, V. Understanding and combating elder abuse in hispanic communities. *J. Elder Abuse Negl.* **1998**, *9*, 5–16. [CrossRef]
6. Xakellis, G.; Brangman, S.A.; Hinton, W.L.; Jones, V.Y.; Masterman, D.; Pan, C.X.; Rivero, J.; Wallhagen, M.; Yeo, G. Curricular framework: Core competencies in multicultural geriatric care. *J. Am. Geriat. Soc.* **2004**, *52*, 137–142. [CrossRef] [PubMed]
7. Evans, K.H.; Bereknyei, S.; Yeo, G.; Hikoyeda, N.; Tzuang, M.; Braddock, C.H. The impact of a faculty development program in health literacy and ethnogeriatrics. *Acad. Med.* **2014**, *89*, 1640–1644. [CrossRef] [PubMed]
8. Velayudhan, L.; Ryu, S.H.; Raczek, M.; Philpot, M.; Lindesay, J.; Critchfield, M.; Livingston, G. Review of brief cognitive tests for patients with suspected dementia. *Int. Psychogeriatr.* **2014**, *26*, 1247–1262. [CrossRef] [PubMed]
9. Jones, R.N.; Gallo, J.J. Education bias in the mini-mental state examination. *Int. Psychogeriatr.* **2001**, *13*, 299–310. [CrossRef] [PubMed]
10. Tombaugh, T.N.; McIntyre, N.J. The mini-mental state examination: A comprehensive review. *J. Am. Geriat. Soc.* **1992**, *40*, 922–935. [CrossRef] [PubMed]
11. Du, Y.; Xu, Q. Health disparities and delayed health care among older adults in california: A perspective from race, ethnicity, and immigration. *Public Health Nurs.* **2016**, *33*, 383–394. [CrossRef]
12. Harris, M.F. Access to preventive care by immigrant populations. *BMC Med.* **2012**, *10*, 55. [CrossRef]
13. *National Standards for Culturally and Linguistically Appropriate Services (clas) in Health and Health Care*; U.S. Department of Health and Human Services Office of Minority Health: Washington, DC, USA, 2013.
14. Chen, A.H.; Youdelman, M.K.; Brooks, J. The legal framework for language access in healthcare settings: Title vi and beyond. *J. Gen. Intern. Med.* **2007**, *22* (Suppl. 2), 362–367. [CrossRef]
15. Plejert, C.; Antelius, E.; Yazdanpanah, M.; Nielsen, T.R. There's a letter called ef' on challenges and repair in interpreter-mediated tests of cognitive functioning in dementia evaluations: A case study. *J. Cross Cult. Gerontol.* **2015**, *30*, 163–187. [CrossRef] [PubMed]
16. Divi, C.; Koss, R.G.; Schmaltz, S.P.; Loeb, J.M. Language proficiency and adverse events in us hospitals: A pilot study. *Int. J. Qual. Health Care* **2007**, *19*, 60–67. [CrossRef] [PubMed]
17. Tamura-Lis, W. Teach-back for quality education and patient safety. *Urol. Nurs.* **2013**, *33*, 267–271, 298. [CrossRef] [PubMed]
18. Chesser, A.K.; Keene Woods, N.; Smothers, K.; Rogers, N. Health literacy and older adults: A systematic review. *Gerontol. Geriat. Med.* **2016**, *2*, 2333721416630492. [CrossRef] [PubMed]
19. Wolf, M.S.; Feinglass, J.; Thompson, J.; Baker, D.W. In search of 'low health literacy': Threshold vs. Gradient effect of literacy on health status and mortality. *Soc. Sci. Med.* **2010**, *70*, 1335–1341. [CrossRef] [PubMed]
20. McDougall, G.J.; Mackert, M.; Becker, H. Memory performance, health literacy, and instrumental activities of daily living of community residing older adults. *Nurs. Res.* **2012**, *61*, 70–75. [CrossRef] [PubMed]
21. Parker, R. Health literacy: A challenge for american patients and their health care providers. *Health Promot. Int.* **2000**, *15*, 277–283. [CrossRef]
22. Berry, J.W. Immigration, acculturation, and adaptation. *Appl. Psychol.* **1997**, *46*, 5–34. [CrossRef]
23. Alegria, M. The challenge of acculturation measures: What are we missing? A commentary on thomson & hoffman-goetz. *Soc. Sci. Med.* **2009**, *69*, 996–998.

24. Fayers, P.M.; Sprangers, M.A. Understanding self-rated health. *Lancet* **2002**, *359*, 187–188. [CrossRef]
25. Lommel, L.L.; Chen, J.L. The relationship between self-rated health and acculturation in hispanic and asian adult immigrants: A systematic review. *J. Immigr. Minor. Health* **2016**, *18*, 468–478. [CrossRef] [PubMed]
26. TD, M. Perceptions of depression and access to mental health care among latino immigrants: Looking beyond one size fits all. *Qual. Health Res.* **2016**, *26*, 1289–1302.
27. Kleinman, A. Culture and depression. *N. Engl. J. Med.* **2004**, *351*, 951–953. [CrossRef] [PubMed]
28. Kleinman, A. Anthropology and psychiatry. The role of culture in cross-cultural research on illness. *Br. J. Psychiatry* **1987**, *151*, 447–454. [CrossRef] [PubMed]
29. Teut, M.; Besch, F.; Witt, C.M.; Stockigt, B. Perceived outcomes of spiritual healing: Results from a prospective case series. *Complement. Med. Res.* **2019**, 1–11. [CrossRef] [PubMed]
30. Hoff, W. Traditional healers and community health. *World Health Forum* **1992**, *13*, 182–187. [PubMed]
31. Prince, M.; Bryce, R.; Albanese, E.; Wimo, A.; Ribeiro, W.; Ferri, C.P. The global prevalence of dementia: A systematic review and metaanalysis. *Alzheimers Dement.* **2013**, *9*, 63–75.e62. [CrossRef] [PubMed]
32. Casas, R.; Guzmán-Vélez, E.; Cardona-Rodriguez, J.; Rodriguez, N.; Quiñones, G.; Izaguirre, B.; Tranel, D. Interpreter-mediated neuropsychological testing of monolingual spanish speakers. *Clin. Neuropsychol.* **2012**, *26*, 88–101. [CrossRef]
33. Goudsmit, M.; van Campen, J.; Schilt, T.; Hinnen, C.; Franzen, S.; Schmand, B. One size does not fit all: Comparative diagnostic accuracy of the rowland universal dementia assessment scale and the mini mental state examination in a memory clinic population with very low education. *Dement. Geriat. Cogn. Dis. Extra* **2018**, *8*, 290–305. [CrossRef]
34. Meagher, J.; Leonard, M.; Donoghue, L.; O'Regan, N.; Timmons, S.; Exton, C.; Cullen, W.; Dunne, C.; Adamis, D.; Maclullich, A.J.; et al. Months backward test: A review of its use in clinical studies. *World J. Psychiatry* **2015**, *5*, 305–314. [CrossRef]
35. Resource Language Translations for Medical Professionals. Available online: https://www.icudelirium.org/medical-professionals/downloads/resource-language-translations (accessed on 11 May 2019).
36. Aranda, M.P. Depression-related disparities among older, low-acculturated U.S. Latinos. *Psychiatr. Times* **2013**, *30*, 1–4.
37. Reuland, D.S.; Cherrington, A.; Watkins, G.S.; Bradford, D.W.; Blanco, R.A.; Gaynes, B.N. Diagnostic accuracy of spanish language depression-screening instruments. *Ann. Fam. Med.* **2009**, *7*, 455–462. [CrossRef] [PubMed]
38. Limon, F.J.; Lamson, A.L.; Hodgson, J.; Bowler, M.; Saeed, S. Screening for depression in latino immigrants: A systematic review of depression screening instruments translated into spanish. *J. Immigr. Minor. Health* **2016**, *18*, 787–798. [CrossRef] [PubMed]
39. Camacho, D.; Estrada, E.; Lagomasino, I.T.; Aranda, M.P.; Green, J. Descriptions of depression and depression treatment in older hispanic immigrants in a geriatric collaborative care program. *Aging Ment. Health* **2018**, *22*, 1050–1056. [CrossRef] [PubMed]
40. Pandav, R.; Fillenbaum, G.; Ratcliff, G.; Dodge, H.; Ganguli, M. Sensitivity and specificity of cognitive and functional screening instruments for dementia: The indo-u.S. Dementia epidemiology study. *J. Am. Geriat. Soc.* **2002**, *50*, 554–561. [CrossRef] [PubMed]
41. Morris, J.C. Clinical dementia rating: A reliable and valid diagnostic and staging measure for dementia of the alzheimer type. *Int. Psychogeriatr.* **1997**, *9* (Suppl. 1), 173–176. [CrossRef] [PubMed]
42. Fillenbaum, G.G.; Chandra, V.; Ganguli, M.; Pandav, R.; Gilby, J.E.; Seaberg, E.C.; Belle, S.; Baker, C.; Echement, D.A.; Nath, L.M. Development of an activities of daily living scale to screen for dementia in an illiterate rural older population in India. *Age Ageing* **1999**, *28*, 161–168. [CrossRef]
43. Suurmond, J.; Seeleman, C. Shared decision-making in an intercultural context. Barriers in the interaction between physicians and immigrant patients. *Patient Educ. Couns.* **2006**, *60*, 253–259. [CrossRef]
44. Acierno, R.; Hernandez, M.A.; Amstadter, A.B.; Resnick, H.S.; Steve, K.; Muzzy, W.; Kilpatrick, D.G. Prevalence and correlates of emotional, physical, sexual, and financial abuse and potential neglect in the united states: The national elder mistreatment study. *Am. J. Public Health* **2010**, *100*, 292–297. [CrossRef]

© 2019 by the authors. Licensee MDPI, Basel, Switzerland. This article is an open access article distributed under the terms and conditions of the Creative Commons Attribution (CC BY) license (http://creativecommons.org/licenses/by/4.0/).

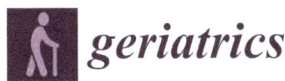

Article

Point of Care Quantitative Assessment of Muscle Health in Older Individuals: An Investigation of Quantitative Muscle Ultrasound and Electrical Impedance Myography Techniques

Lisa D Hobson-Webb [1,*], Paul J Zwelling [1], Ashley N Pifer [1], Carrie M Killelea [2,3], Mallory S Faherty [2,3], Timothy C Sell [2,3] and Amy M Pastva [2,4]

1. Duke University Department of Neurology/Neuromuscular Division, Durham, NC 27710, USA; paul.zwelling@duke.edu (P.J.Z.); ashley.pifer@duke.edu (A.N.P.)
2. Duke University Department of Orthopaedic Surgery, Durham, NC 27710, USA; carolyn.killelea@duke.edu (C.M.K.); mallory.faherty@duke.edu (M.S.F.); tcs30@duke.edu (T.C.S.); amy.pastva@duke.edu (A.M.P.)
3. Michael W. Krzyzewski Human Performance Laboratory, Durham, NC 27710, USA
4. Duke University Claude D. Pepper Older American Independence Center Durham, NC 27710, USA
* Correspondence: lisa.hobsonwebb@duke.edu; Tel.: +01-919-668-2277

Received: 28 November 2018; Accepted: 13 December 2018; Published: 16 December 2018

Abstract: *Background:* Muscle health is recognized for its critical role in the functionality and well-being of older adults. Readily accessible, reliable, and inexpensive methods of measuring muscle health are needed to advance research and clinical care. *Methods:* In this prospective, blinded study, 27 patients underwent quantitative muscle ultrasound (QMUS), standard electrical impedance myography (sEIM), and handheld electrical impedance myography (hEIM) of the anterior thigh musculature by two independent examiners. Subjects also had dual-energy X-ray absorptiometry (DEXA) scans and standardized tests of physical function and strength. Data were analyzed for intra- and inter-rater reliability, along with correlations with DEXA and physical measures. *Results:* Measures of intra- and inter-rater reliability were excellent (>0.90) for all QMUS, sEIM, and hEIM parameters except intra-rater reliability of rectus femoris echointensity (0.87–0.89). There were moderate, inverse correlations between QMUS, sEIM, and hEIM parameters and measures of knee extensor strength. Moderate to strong correlations (0.57–0.81) were noted between investigational measures and DEXA-measured fat mass. *Conclusions:* QMUS, sEIM and hEIM were highly reliable in a controlled, same-day testing protocol. Multiple correlations with measures of strength and body composition were noted for each method. Point-of-care technologies may provide an alternative means of measuring health.

Keywords: elderly; aging; muscle; ultrasound; electrical impedance myography; point of care; TUG; frailty

1. Introduction

Muscle health is recognized for its critical role in the well-being and functionality of older adults [1]. Aging is associated with loss of muscle mass, known as sarcopenia, and loss of muscle quality, manifesting as replacement of healthy muscle tissue by adipose and water. Both have been associated with limitations in physical activity and function, including the performance of routine activities of daily required for independent living [2,3]. To date, muscle health assessment has primarily focused on muscle quantity; however, this assessment alone may overestimate the amount of functional muscle. Computed tomography (CT), magnetic resonance imaging (MRI), and dual energy X-ray absorptiometry (DEXA) scans are gold standard measures used to assess the quantity and quality of muscle [4]. CT has most frequently been used to assess fatty infiltration of muscle, which manifests as a reduced attenuation coefficient [5]. However, given that these scans are expensive, not readily accessible in the outpatient or community setting, or well-suited for home use, there is a need for novel means of measuring muscle health for both clinical and research purposes.

Ultrasound provides a rapid, non-invasive, portable and inexpensive means of evaluating muscle. Although new approaches, including shear wave elastography, are being investigated, measures of muscle size and signal are traditionally used. Muscle size is often expressed as thickness or cross-sectional area of the muscle, while signal is described in terms of echointensity (EI). As expected, reduced muscle size at select sites has been linked to an overall reduction in muscle mass. Studied primarily in disease states, elevated EI represents increased intramuscular fibrous composition and generally correlates with worsening muscle health [6]. Other factors that can affect EI include ultrasound system settings, aging, sex and level of conditioning, making its interpretation somewhat challenging [7,8].

A number of recent studies have explored the role of quantitative muscle ultrasound (QMUS) in the critically ill, but less is known about the role of muscle health in community-dwelling elderly individuals [9,10]. An early study of 92 elderly Japanese patients demonstrated moderate inverse correlations between EI and quadriceps strength among middle-aged and elderly individuals, independent of age or muscle thickness [11]. More recently, Mirón Mombiela et al. examined EI as biomarker of frailty in a study of patients aged 20 to 90 years [12]. The group found, similar to the aforementioned study, moderate, inverse correlations between EI and quadriceps strength. Higher EI values were also associated with greater frailty.

Electrical impedance myography (EIM) is another technology receiving recent attention for measurement of muscle health. Differing EIM devices are available, but the basic principle is that these systems measure the muscle impedance to flow of a painless, electrical current. Impedance is not very high in healthy muscle but is known to increase in conditions that impact normal muscle architecture [13]. Prior studies in amyotrophic lateral sclerosis (ALS) and Duchenne muscular dystrophy (DMD) demonstrate the promise of this technique [14–16]. Unlike imaging studies, EIM can be performed with little training. It is portable and hand-held devices are available. The equipment is inexpensive; some consumer-marketed devices are available for less than US $100. These advantages are appealing, but data on reliability, longitudinal change, correlation with established measures of strength, and the impact of patient positioning, hydration and many other factors are lacking.

Given the need for improved muscle health data and the advantages of QMUS and EIM, the current study was designed to investigate the feasibility of using both technologies in the community-dwelling elderly. The aims of the current study were to determine the inter-rater reliability and reproducibility of QMUS and EIM. In addition, we examined the correlations between QMUS, EIM and currently accepted measures of physical strength, physical function, and muscle mass. The findings demonstrate that both QMUS and EIM are reliable tools that correlate with functional and DEXA measures.

2. Materials and Methods

2.1. Research Cohort

The Duke Institutional Review Board approved the current study (Duke IRB Protocol 00076633). Twenty-seven subjects were recruited through use of the Pepper Center (Duke IRB Protocol 00016209)/Duke Aging Center Subject Registry (Duke IRB Pro00005016) from January to December 2017. Subjects were recruited through letters sent to individuals that had previously consented to being listed in the Duke Aging Center Subject Registry. Flyers were also posted at geriatric clinics and in physical therapy clinics around campus. Interested subjects replied to the study coordinator to learn more about the study before the informed consent process took place.

Inclusion criteria were age >65 years and the ability to provide informed consent. Those unable to provide informed consent were excluded. Patients with known active malignancy, myositis, motor neuron disease, inability to ambulate independently or taking daily steroids were also excluded as these factors can affect muscle bulk rapidly.

Upon providing informed consent to participate in the study, subjects underwent testing (estimated time involvement 3–4 h) over 1–2 site visits. All study activities were completed within a 7-day period. QMUS and EIM were performed on the same day for all patients studied.

2.2. Investigational Techniques

2.2.1. Quantitative Muscle Ultrasonography (QMUS)

QMUS of the right rectus femoris and vastus intermedius complex was performed at one-third the distance between the patella and anterior superior iliac spine. The subject was positioned at rest in the supine position with the knee in passive extension. Two independent examiners (LHW, PJZ) each collected three separate images at this site. LHW is a neurologist with 14 years of experience in neuromuscular ultrasound, while PJZ is an electrodiagnostic technician trained to perform muscle ultrasound for the purpose of the current study. PJZ had 2 weeks of training prior to study initiation, provided by LHW. The examiners were blinded to the results of each other's imaging and other study results.

A Esaote MyLabSIX Ultrasound system was used, equipped with a 6–18 MHz linear array probe. Probe frequency was held at 6 MHz with constant gain, compression, and time gain compensation settings. Depth was adjusted as needed to accommodate the size of the patient imaged. Ultrasound data were digitally stored in the ultrasound system and processed off-line after each subject's visit was complete.

Both examiners performed off-line independent, analysis of images. Subcutaneous fat thickness was calculated by measuring the distance from the skin surface to the superficial fascia of the muscles using on-screen calipers. Thickness of the rectus femoris and vastus intermedius was then measured in a similar manner using the femoral border and muscle fascia as landmarks. EI was measured by exporting the still images to Adobe Photoshop (Adobe Systems Incorporated, San Jose, CA, USA) for gray scale analysis scoring. The gray scale ranges from 0 to 255 (0 = black, 255 = white). A region of interest (ROI) was drawn as large as possible for each muscle, making effort to exclude fascial borders, bone and any artifact present in the image. As each examiner generated three measurements for each parameter recorded, the mean was calculated for thickness, while the mean, standard deviation, and median were calculated for gray scale scoring.

2.2.2. Electrical Impedance Myography (EIM)—Standard Equipment (sEIM)

sEIM was performed over the right rectus femoris/vastus intermedius complex, as outlined in the QMUS section. sEIM was conducted with a device (SFB7 Impedimed, Inc., Pinkenba, Australia) previously used in the assessment of neuromuscular disease. The device provides a painless, surface alternating current over muscle with four adhesive electrodes placed across the muscle for recording. Measurements were taken over the muscles' axial plane, which is the accepted standard. Three measures each of resistance (R) and reactance (Xc) and phase (θ) were recorded for each muscle at 50 kHz and 200 kHz then averaged for the mean value of each. The subjects had sEIM performed by two independent examiners (LHW, PJZ), creating two complete sets of measures. Neither examiner had experience with this device prior to the current study and were self-trained using the company provided instructional materials. The examiners were blinded to the results of each other's testing and other study results.

2.2.3. Electrical Impedance Myography (hEIM)-Handheld Device

A handheld, portable, commercially available fitness tracker device was used (Chisel, Skulpt, Inc., San Franscisco, CA, USA). This smart-phone sized device uses the same methods as previously described for sEIM but has incorporated fixed electrodes and provides users with both a body fat measurement for each muscle assessed, as well as a Muscle Quality (MQ) score derived from raw EIM data. The frequencies used with the handheld system are proprietary and cannot be selected or altered by the user. MQ is derived from resistance and reactance measures, but the values are not available on the commercial display. The MQ scale ranges from 0 to 100, with 100 being the best score possible. The scoring system is as follows: 0–20 Needs Work, 20–40 Good, 60–80 Fit, and 80–100 Athletic.

The hEIM electrodes on the device were moistened with water and then placed over the right rectus femoris/vastus intermedius complex for approximately 5 s, while measurements were made. The subjects had three hEIM measurements performed by two independent clinicians (LHW, PJZ). Neither examiner had experience with this device prior to the current study and were self-trained using the company provided instructional materials. The examiners were blinded to the results of each other's testing and other study results.

2.2.4. Standard Clinical Measures

Age, sex, height, and weight were recorded for each subject on the day of their first study visit.

2.2.5. Lower Extremity Strength and Physical Function Testing

Quantitative testing of lower extremity strength was performed by personnel at the Duke Sports Science Institute's Michael W. Krzyzewski Human Performance Lab, under the direction of authors (AMP, TCS, MSF, CMK). Personnel were blinded to other study results.

An isokinetic dynamometer (Biodex System 3 Multi-Joint Testing and Rehabilitation System, White Plains, NY, USA) was used to measure leg strength and data were assessed using the system's proprietary software. The test protocol was maintained for all subjects as follows: concentric (CON) at $180°/s$ and isometric (ISO) at $0°/s$ at a ~$60°$ knee angle. Subjects were placed in a comfortable, seated position on the Biodex System 3 chair and secured using thigh, pelvic and torso straps in order to minimize accessory body movements and isolate performance at the knee. The lateral femoral epicondyle was used as the bony landmark for aligning the axis of rotation of the knee joint with the axis of rotation of the dynamometer axis. Subjects were provided a warm-up session of three repetitions at 50% of maximum effort and three repetitions at 100% of maximum effort for both the ISO and CON tests. A one-minute rest period was provided prior to the actual testing and between the two different test modes (ISO and CON). Subjects were instructed to give maximum effort throughout the entire test. For the CON test, five maximal quadriceps contractions at $180°/s$ were performed. For the ISO test, the leg was flexed to $60°$. Subjects completed five repetitions (5-s hold for each rep) with 10 s of rest between repetitions. The Timed Up and Go test (TUG) was included as a standardized and validated physical function task measure in older adults. The test measures the time taken to arise from a chair, walk three meters, turn around, walk back to the chair, and sit down.

2.2.6. Imaging Studies

Whole-body dual energy X-ray absorptiometry (DEXA) was performed on all subjects and considered to be the gold standard for muscle mass and fat calculations of the proximal right lower extremity (thigh). Staff radiologists blinded to other study results interpreted the DEXA scans.

2.3. Data Analysis

Study data were collected and managed using REDCap electronic data capture tools hosted at Duke University. REDCap (Research Electronic Data Capture) is a secure, web-based application designed to support data capture for research studies, providing (1) an intuitive interface for validated data entry; (2) audit trails for tracking data manipulation and export procedures; (3) automated export procedures for seamless data downloads to common statistical packages; and (4) procedures for importing data from external sources.

QMUS and EIM measures were analyzed for inter-rater reliability as measured by the InterClass correlation. Intra-rater reliability was also assessed. For QMUS, muscle thickness, subcutaneous fat thickness and muscle EI were examined for correlation with patient demographics, DEXA measures of muscle mass, and the results of isokinetic and isometric testing. For sEIM, the impedance measures were analyzed for correlation with the same set of clinical measures. For the hEIM, the correlation between clinical measures and both the MQ score and muscle fat percentage were assessed.

Statistical significance was set at $p \leq 0.05$, while a trend is defined as $p = 0.051–0.10$.

3. Results

Twenty-seven volunteers were recruited and enrolled for the study. No participants were excluded upon contact with the study coordinator. The cohort was 70% male with mean age of 72.6 years. More detailed demographics and details on the absolute QMUS values are shown in Table 1. For each subject, all testing was completed within a 7-day window. QMUS and EIM were always performed on the same day and examiner 1 and 2's measurements were separated by a period of at least 15 min.

Table 1. Subject demographics and group quantitative muscle ultrasound (QMUS) results.

Male/Female	19 (70%)/8 (30%)
Age (years)	72.6 ± 5 (range 65–82 years)
Height (cm)	172.2 ± 11 (range 152–200 cm)
Weight (kg)	83.3 kg ± 19 (range 52–131 kg)
BMI (kg/m^2)	28.1
Ultrasound Measurements	
Fat thickness (mm)	8.8 ± 7 (range 0.6–23.5)
RF thickness (mm)	13.7 ± 6 (range 1.2–23.5)
VI thickness (mm)	13.2 ± 6 (range 0.9–22.7)
Echointensity RF	94.16 ± 20 (range 68.8–167.5)
VI	62.6 ± 32 (range 10.3–121.2)

3.1. Intra- and Inter-Rater Reliability

Intra-and inter-rater reliability data for all investigational techniques are summarized in Table 2.

Table 2. Intra- and inter-rater reliability.

Test	Intra-Rater		Inter-Rater
	Examiner 1	Examiner 2	
QMUS			
SQ thickness	0.98 *	0.99 *	0.99 *
RF thickness	0.98 *	0.98 *	0.98 *
VI thickness	0.98 *	0.99 *	0.97 *
RF echointensity	0.89 *	0.87 *	0.94 *
VI echointensity	0.93 *	0.93 *	0.96 **
sEIM			
50 kHz R	1.0 *	1.0 *	1.0 *
50 kHz Xc	1.0 *	1.0 *	0.99 *
50 kHz θ	1.0 *	0.99 *	0.99 *
200 kHz R	1.0 *	1.0 *	1.0 *
200 kHz Xc	1.0 *	0.99 *	0.99 *
200 kHz θ	0.97 *	0.99 *	0.98 *
hEIM			
Fat %	0.99 *	0.99 *	0.98 *
Muscle Quality	0.99 *	0.99 *	0.98 *

hEIM: handheld electrical impedance myography; Hz: hertz; QMUS: quantitative muscle ultrasound; R: resistance; RF: rectus femoris; sEIM: standard electrical impedance myography; SQ: subcutaneous tissue; VI: vastus intermedius; Xc: reactance; θ = phase; *: $p < 0.0001$; **: $p = 0.005$.

3.1.1. QMUS

Intra-rater reliability for subcutaneous fat thickness was excellent ($r = 0.98$, $p < 0.0001$ for examiner 1 and $r = 0.99$, $p < 0.0001$ for examiner 2). Rectus femoris thickness reliability was high for both examiners ($r = 0.98$, $p < 0.0001$). Vastus intermedius thickness had good agreement ($r = 0.98$, $p < 0.0001$ for examiner 1 and $r = 0.99$, $p < 0.0001$ for examiner 2). Intra-rater reliability for rectus femoris echointensity was high for both examiners ($r = 0.89$, $p < 0.0001$ for examiner 1 and $r = 0.87$, $p < 0.0001$ for examiner 2). For vastus intermedius echointensity, intra-rater agreement was similar ($r = 0.93$, $p < 0.0001$ for examiner 1 and $r = 0.93$, $p < 0.0001$ for examiner 2).

Inter-rater reliability for subcutaneous fat thickness was excellent ($r = 0.99$, $p < 0.0001$). Rectus femoris and vastus intermedius thickness demonstrated similar results ($r = 0.98$, $p < 0.0001$ and $r = 0.97$, $p < 0.0001$, respectively). Unexpectedly, mean muscle echointensity measures for vastus intermedius had excellent agreement ($r = 0.96$, $p = 0.005$), as did rectus femoris ($r = 0.94$, $p < 0.0001$).

No significant differences between examiners were found for any QMUS parameter.

3.1.2. sEIM

Intra-rater reliability measures were extremely high for 50 kHz, which was not unexpected as all measures occurred within a one-second-measurement period that required no movement of electrodes. Examiner 1 performed well for R, Xc and θ. ($r = 1.0$, $p < 0.0001$). For examiner 2, R and Xc had extraordinary reliability ($r = 1.0$, $p < 0.0001$), with θ performing only slightly worse ($r = 0.99$, $p < 0.0001$). Examiner 1 intra-rater reliability at 200 kHz was the same for R and Xc ($r = 1.0$, $p < 0.0001$). There was slightly lower agreement for θ ($r = 0.97$, $p < 0.0001$) that appeared to be secondary to a single outlying value related to patient movement. For examiner 2, reliability was also high for R ($r = 1.0$, $p < 0.0001$), Xc ($r = 0.99$, $p < 0.0001$) and θ ($r = 0.99$, $p < 0.0001$).

Inter-rater measurements were separated by several minutes, but performed well. The 50-kHz sEIM had excellent inter-rater reliability for R ($r = 1.0$, $p < 0.0001$), Xc ($r = 0.99$, $p < 0.0001$) and θ ($r = 0.99$, $p < 0.0001$). For 200 Hz, measures were similar for R ($r = 1.0$, $p < 0.0001$), Xc ($r = 0.99$, $p < 0.0001$) and θ ($r = 0.98$, $p < 0.0001$). Please note that a single data point from subject 1, examiner 1 200 kHz Xc was excluded due to a data entry error and concerns over accuracy.

No significant differences were found between examiners for any sEIM parameter at either 50 or 200 kHz.

3.1.3. hEIM

hEIM performed well on intra-rater reliability measures. Examiner 1 performed well on muscle quality ($r = 0.99$, $p < 0.0001$) and muscle fat % ($r = 0.99$, $p < 0.0001$). Examiner 2 did just as well for muscle quality ($r = 0.99$, $p < 0.0001$) and muscle fat % ($r = 0.99$, $p < 0.0001$). Inter-rater reliability for muscle quality was excellent ($r = 0.98$, $p < 0.0001$), as was muscle fat % ($r = 0.98$, $p < 0.0001$). It is not surprising that the reliability was essentially identical for the two measures, given that they are inter-related and reported simultaneously. No significant differences were found between examiners for hEIM-measured muscle quality or muscle fat %.

3.2. Correlations

Detailed information on all correlations between investigational measures can be found in Tables 3 and 4.

Table 3. Correlations between test results and functional measures.

Test	Isometric Normalized Peak Torque	Isokinetic Normalized Peak Torque	Timed Up and Go (TUG)
QMUS			
SQ thickness	$-0.56, p = 0.002$	$-0.50, p = 0.08$	—
RF thickness	—	—	$-0.37, p = 0.06$
VI thickness	—	—	—
RF echointensity	$-0.48, p = 0.01$	—	—
VI echointensity	—	—	—
sEIM			
50 kHz R	$-0.46, p = 0.016$	—	—
50 kHz Xc	—	—	—
50 kHz θ	$-0.45, p = 0.02$	—	$0.35, p = 0.07$
200 kHz R	$-0.57, p = 0.01$	$-0.53, p = 0.01$	$0.45, p = 0.04$
200 kHz Xc	—	—	—
200 kHz θ	$-0.54, p = 0.01$	$-0.51, p = 0.02$	$0.49, p = 0.02$
50/200 kHz θ Ratio	—	—	—
200/50 kHz Phase Ratio	$0.50, p = 0.01$	$0.44, p = 0.027$	—
hEIM			
Fat %	$-0.49, p = 0.009$	—	—
Muscle Quality	—	—	—
DEXA			
Thigh muscle mass	—	—	—
Thigh fat mass	$-0.52, p = 0.005$	$-0.39, p = 0.04$	—

hEIM: handheld electrical impedance myography; Hz: hertz; QMUS: quantitative muscle ultrasound; R: resistance; RF: rectus femoris; sEIM: standard electrical impedance myography; SQ: subcutaneous tissue; VI: vastus intermedius; Xc: reactance; θ: phase; —: no significant correlations observed.

Table 4. Correlations between investigational tests and DEXA results.

Test	DEXA-Measured Right Thigh Fat Mass	DEXA-Measured Right Thigh Muscle Mass
QMUS		
SQ thickness	0.81, $p < 0.0001$	—
RF thickness	—	0.53, $p = 0.0045$
VI thickness	—	0.54, $p = 0.004$
RF echointensity	0.35, $p = 0.07$	−0.33, $p = 0.09$
VI echointensity	—	−0.52, $p = 0.006$
sEIM		
50 kHz R	0.65, $p = 0.0003$	—
50 kHz Xc	—	—
50 kHz θ	0.57, $p = 0.002$	−0.37, $p = 0.06$
200 kHz R	0.70, $p < 0.0001$	−0.26, $p = 0.06$
200 kHz Xc	—	−0.46, $p = 0.016$
200 kHz θ	0.72, $p < 0.001$	−0.34, $p = 0.09$
50/200 kHz θ Ratio	—	—
200/50 kHz θ Ratio	−0.41, $p = 0.041$	—
hEIM		
Fat %	0.74, $p < 0.0001$	−0.38, $p = 0.0492$
Muscle Quality	−0.72, $p < 0.0001$	—

hEIM: handheld electrical impedance myography; Hz: hertz; QMUS: quantitative muscle ultrasound; R: resistance; RF: rectus femoris; sEIM: standard electrical impedance myography; SQ: subcutaneous tissue; VI: vastus intermedius; Xc: capacitance; θ; phase; —: no significant correlations observed.

3.2.1. QMUS

Rectus femoris and vastus intermedius thickness did not correlate with isokinetic normalized peak torque. However, there was a negative correlation with subcutaneous fat thickness ($r = -0.50$, $p = 0.008$). The same pattern was evident for isometric normalized peak torque, with an inverse correlation present for subcutaneous fat thickness ($r = -0.56$, $p = 0.002$). TUG time trended toward a correlation with rectus femoris thickness ($r = -0.37$, $p = 0.06$), but there were no correlations with vastus intermedius or subcutaneous fat thickness.

Rectus femoris thickness correlated with DEXA measured right thigh muscle mass ($r = 0.53$, $p = 0.0045$), as did vastus intermedius thickness ($r = 0.54$, $p = 0.004$). There was no correlation observed with subcutaneous fat thickness. For DEXA measured right thigh fat mass, there was a strong correlation with subcutaneous fat thickness ($r = 0.81$, $p < 0.0001$). There were no correlations between DEXA measured right thigh fat mass and muscle thickness.

Muscle echointensity measures were also analyzed. Rectus femoris echointensity did not correlate with isokinetic normalized peak torque or TUG time, but did inversely correlate with isometric normalized peak torque ($r = -0.48$, $p = 0.01$). Vastus intermedius echointensity did not correlate with isokinetic normalized peak torque, isometric peak torque or TUG time. There was a trend between rectus femoris echointensity and DEXA-measured fat mass of the right leg ($r = 0.35$, $p = 0.07$) that was not seen for vastus intermedius. Similarly, a trend toward an inverse correlation between rectus femoris echointensity and DEXA-measured muscle mass of the right thigh was present ($r = -0.33$, $p = 0.09$). In addition, there was an inverse correlation between vastus intermedius echointensity and DEXA-measured muscle mass of the right thigh ($r = -0.52$, $p = 0.006$)

3.2.2. sEIM

At 50 kHz, moderate negative correlations were noted between isometric normalized peak torque of knee extension and R ($r = -0.46$, $p = 0.016$) and phase ($r = -0.45$, $p = 0.02$), but not for Xc. No correlations were observed between the 50 kHz measures and isokinetic normalized peak torque of knee extension. No significant correlations were found between the 50 kHz measures and TUG time, although a trend was seen for θ ($r = 0.35$, $p = 0.07$).

For DEXA measured right leg muscle mass and 50 kHz measures, there was a trend toward a negative correlation with θ ($r = -0.37$, $p = 0.06$), but not for R or Xc. For right leg fat mass, there were correlations with R ($r = 0.65$, $p = 0.0003$) and θ ($r = 0.57$, $p = 0.002$), but not Xc.

At 200 kHz, negative correlations were again noted between isometric normalized peak torque of knee extension and R ($r=-0.57$, $p = 0.01$), as well as θ ($r = -0.54$, $p = 0.01$), but not Xc. There were also negative correlations with isokinetic normalized peak torque of knee extension and R ($r = -0.53$, $p = 0.01$), as well as θ ($r = -0.51$, $p = 0.02$). There was no correlation between Xc and isokinetic normalized peak torque of the anterior quadriceps. For TUG time, there was a positive correlation with R ($r = 0.45$, $p = 0.04$) and θ ($r = 0.49$, $p = 0.02$), but not Xc.

For DEXA measured right leg muscle mass and 200 kHz measures, there was a moderate negative correlation with Xc ($r = -0.46$, $p = 0.016$). There was a trend toward a negative correlation with R ($r = -0.26$, $p = 0.06$) and θ ($r = -0.34$, $p = 0.09$). For right leg fat mass, there were correlations with R ($r = 0.70$, $p < 0.0001$) and θ ($r = 0.72$, $p < 0.001$), but not Xc.

Use of the 50/200 kHz phase ratio negated all correlations, while a 200/50 kHz θ ratio gave nearly identical results to the 50 and 200 kHz measures for correlation with functional testing (Table 3) but performed worse for correlation with DEXA-estimated thigh fat and muscle mass.

Based upon these observations, the 200 kHz setting correlated best with measures of physical function and body composition.

3.2.3. hEIM

There was no correlation between isokinetic normalized peak torque of the quadriceps and either MQ or muscle fat %. For isometric normalized peak torque, there was an inverse correlation with muscle fat % ($r = -0.49$, $p = 0.009$). TUG time did not correlate with either parameter.

MQ did not correlate with DEXA-measured muscle mass of the right thigh but had a strong inverse correlation with fat mass ($r = -0.72$, $p < 0.0001$). Muscle fat % had a strong correlation with DEXA-measured fat mass of the thigh ($r = 0.74$, $p < 0.0001$) and a weaker inverse correlation with muscle mass ($r = -0.38$, $p = 0.0492$).

3.2.4. DEXA Correlation with Strength and Functional Measures

DEXA-measured muscle mass did not correlate with isometric normalized peak torque, isokinetic normalized peak torque or TUG time. DEXA-measured thigh fat mass had moderate, negative correlations with both isometric ($r = -0.52$, $p = 0.005$) and isokinetic ($r = -0.39$, $p = 0.04$) normalized peak torque, but not TUG time.

Of little surprise, isometric and isokinetic normalized peak torque correlated with TUG time ($r = -0.61$, $p = 0.001$; $r = -0.37$, $p = 0.01$).

4. Discussion

In this pilot study, we aimed to determine if QMUS, sEIM or hEIM would be feasible tools for assessing muscle health and function in older adults. Validating each of these techniques first required an assessment of intra- and inter-rater reliability, followed by analysis of correlations with accepted measures of muscle mass, strength, and physical function. The results show that each method was reliable within and between examiners after minimal training and correlated with both DEXA and functional measures. Our study was unique in that it examined intra- and inter-rater agreement and included a mixed population of community dwelling older adults. The population consisted of both men and women; those with chronic medical conditions were not excluded. In the following sections, the results of each investigational technique are analyzed separately and compared with prior literature.

4.1. QMUS

The QMUS portion of our study was unique in that it examined intra- and inter-rater agreement in a mixed population of community dwelling older adults. Subcutaneous fat thickness was also measured, which has not been a focus of prior publications. Additionally, our study compared QMUS results to standard physical rehabilitation-administered strength testing, functional task measures and DEXA scans.

The intra-rater and inter-rater reliability in the current study were excellent for all tissue thickness measures (0.97–0.99). These are very similar to a recent study examining reliability for rectus femoris measurements [17]. Multiple other publications have reported similar results for anterior thigh imaging [18–21]. The intra- and inter-rater agreement for EI in the current study (0.87–0.96) aligned with previous publications. For example, Ishida et al. found an inter-rater reliability of 0.96 for EI of the rectus femoris, while we found a value of 0.94 [17]. Other recent studies have found similar values. These findings provide reassurance that QMUS measures are accurate and repeatable between examinations, as long as the imaging is performed according to a standardized protocol.

In comparing the current QMUS with prior publications, our findings align well with the previously mentioned Fukumoto study of 92 elderly women in regards to patient age, muscle thickness, and EI [11]. This is encouraging when considering the possibility of generalizing results, as the two studies were performed in different patient populations and with different ultrasound systems. The correlations noted between QMUS parameters and strength measurements are also similar.

Lopez et al. examined the relationship between quadriceps echointensity and functional measures in 50 healthy, elderly men [22]. The quadriceps were considered as a group for the purpose of analyzing EI and the mean value was 69.78 ± 11.4, different than seen in the current study (94.16 ± 20 for rectus femoris and 62.6 ± 32 for vastus intermedius). This may reflect the inclusion of only healthy patients, a younger population, lower BMI, the averaging of all quadriceps musculature in calculating the EI and differences in ultrasound systems. Despite the differences in absolute values, the authors found similar, moderate inverse correlations between EI and strength [20].

Similar to other studies [12,22,23], we found that EI correlated better with strength measures than did muscle thickness. In their discussion, Lopez et al. note that the presence of adipose tissue might be more relevant to age-related reductions in strength than the loss of muscle mass alone. Further supporting this hypothesis is our finding that subcutaneous fat thickness had moderate, inverse correlations with muscle strength ($r = -0.50$ to -0.56). This QMUS finding is felt to be accurate, given the strong correlation ($r = 0.81$) with the gold standard DEXA measurement of right thigh fat mass. As QMUS measured subcutaneous fat thickness is much more easily obtained than DEXA measures, QMUS may provide an excellent clinical and research tool for monitoring body fat composition.

4.2. sEIM

sEIM performed extremely well in parameters of intra- and inter-rater reliability (range 0.97–1.0). This was not unexpected given the short interval between trials, the easily accessible muscle chosen for analysis and the standardized protocol. Over the years, different sEIM devices have been assessed, some with fixed electrodes and some using the disposable electrode method described here. A fixed electrode array would be expected to reduce error and improve results.

Both 50 and 200 kHz frequencies were tested in the current study. Most early work focused on use of the 50 kHz frequency in sarcopenia [13]. Aaron et al. 2006 found aging to be associated with reductions in muscle impedance, specifically, the 50-kHz phase, in a cross-sectional study of 100 people [24]. This was most pronounced in men and those over age 60, but only 4 people older than

75 years were included in the study. A follow-up study demonstrated lower 50 kHz reactance, not phase, with aging. Again, men seemed to suffer more decline than women [25].

In our study, moderate, inverse correlations were found between isometric normalized peak torque and both resistance and phase at 50 and 200 kHz (Table 3). The relationship was somewhat stronger for 200 kHz measures, which also displayed similar correlations with normalized isokinetic peak torque. Only the 200 kHz measures had a moderate correlation with TUG time, although a weaker trend was observed for 50 kHz phase.

Good correlations were found between both 50 and 200 kHz resistance and phase with DEXA measured fat mass (Table 4). Again, 200 kHz measures performed better. There were trends toward correlation with muscle mass, but only 200 kHz fat mass reached statistical significance.

4.3. hEIM

To the best of our knowledge, there is only one other published study on the direct-to-consumer hEIM device used here [26]. The purpose of testing the device was to determine if it could be deployed in homes and possibly used by patients and research subjects for longitudinal monitoring of muscle health. No modifications were made to the system and there were no attempts to extract and analyze raw data. Intra-and inter-rater reliability was excellent (0.98–0.99) for muscle quality and % fat as measured by the device. This indicates that with minimal training, the measures are reliable for use in an outpatient clinical setting, warranting larger trials.

hEIM % fat had a moderate inverse correlation with isometric normalized peak torque, but muscle quality's correlation with this measure did not reach clinical significance. There was a strong correlation between hEIM measured % fat and DEXA measured right thigh fat mass (0.74) and a weaker correlation with the TUG time (−0.38). Again, this suggests that increased body and muscle fat have a more profound negative impact on function than muscle mass alone.

The findings here are similar to that found by McLester et al., who studied a population of healthy young adults (mean age 24–25 years). Their study found high agreement between examiners and also found hEIM to be a viable alternative for measuring body fat % [24].

4.4. Study Limitations

The current study is not without limitations and poses new questions. Methodologically, the frequencies used by the hEIM were not available, so a direct comparison between the sEIM and hEIM devices could not be performed. This pilot study had a small sample size ($n = 27$), but a larger cohort would be more likely to strengthen the correlations and trends seen here rather than weaken them. Using multiple muscles, as opposed to a single muscle may alter observed correlations as well. In addition, the study was not powered to detect differences between men and women, which may have been missed in this group. Furthermore, the extremely high reliability seen between examiners is likely related to the strict training provided and the fact that all investigative measures were performed on the same day.

Additional studies are needed to determine the reliability of electrical impedance myography measures over multiple visits, although data by Geisbush et al. suggest high reliability when electrical impedance measurements are separated by 3–7 days [27]. Muscle ultrasound has also demonstrated high reliability when performed on separate days [28]. The effects of hydration, changes in skin impedance and activity prior to testing may affect reliability and should be addressed in future projects. As a final note, the hEIM device was not deployed into subjects' homes to see if they were able to use the device with ease. Future studies will require a lapse of days to weeks prior to determining the real-world reliability of QMUS, sEIM, and hEIM.

5. Conclusions

QMUS, sEIM and hEIM all demonstrated excellent intra- and inter-rater reliability in a controlled, same-day testing protocol. Furthermore, multiple correlations with measures of muscle strength and body composition were noted for each method. Of particular interest is the finding that in older adults, the quality of muscle (i.e., lower % muscle fat) had stronger correlations with strength and function than muscle mass alone. This was true for QMUS, sEIM, and hEIM parameters. DEXA measures of lower extremity fat and muscle mass did not outperform ultrasound or EIM in this regard, suggesting that point-of-care, non-radiating inexpensive technologies may one day replace it as the gold standard.

The current findings require replication and further analysis in larger studies but suggest that interventions to reduce body fat may improve the health of elderly individuals.

Author Contributions: Conceptualization, L.DH.-W. and A.M.P.; Methodology, L.DH.-W. and A.M.P.; Validation, L.DH.-W., P.J.Z., A.N.P., T.C.S., A.M.P.; Formal analysis, L.DH.-W.; Investigation, L.DH.-W., P.J.Z., T.C.S., M.S.F., C.M.K., A.M.P.; Resources, L.DH.-W. and T.C.S.; Data curation, L.DH.-W., A.N.P.; Writing—original draft preparation, L.DH.-W.; Writing—review and editing, L.DH.-W., A.M.P., T.C.S., M.S.F., C.M.K.; Visualization, L.DH.-W.; Supervision, L.DH.-W. and A.M.P.; Project administration, L.DH.-W., P.J.Z., A.N.P, T.C.S., C.M.K., A.M.P.; Funding acquisition, L.DH.-W.

Funding: This research was funded by the National Institute on Aging, Duke Claude D Pepper Older Americans Independence Center, grant number P30 AG028716.

Acknowledgments: The authors would like to acknowledge Kevin Caves and Miriam C. Morey of Duke University for their assistance in designing the current study and ensuring its success.

Conflicts of Interest: The authors declare no conflict of interest. The funders had no role in the design of the study; in the collection, analyses, or interpretation of data; in the writing of the manuscript, or in the decision to publish the results.

References

1. Lauretani, F.; Russo, C.R.; Badinelli, S.; Bartali, B.; Cavazzini, C.; Di Iorio, A.; Corsi, A.M.; Rantanen, T.; Guralnik, J.M.; Ferrucci, L. Age-associated changes in skeletal muscles and their effect on mobility: An operational diagnosis of sarcopenia. *J. Appl. Physiol.* **2003**, *95*, 1851–1860. [CrossRef] [PubMed]
2. Hirani, V.; Blyth, F.; Naganathan, V.; Le Couteur, D.G.; Seibel, M.G.; Waite, M.J.; Handelsman, D.J.; Cumming, R.G. Sarcopenia is associated with incident disability, institutionalization, and mortality in community-dwelling older men: The Concord Health and Ageing in Men Project. *J. Am. Med. Dir. Assoc.* **2015**, *16*, 607–613. [CrossRef] [PubMed]
3. Visser, M.; Goodpaster, B.H.; Kritchevsky, S.B.; Newman, A.B.; Nevitt, M.; Rubin, S.M.; Simonsick, E.M.; Harris, T.B. Muscle mass, muscle strength, and muscle fat infiltration as predictors of incident mobility limitations in well-functioning older persons. *J. Gerontol. A Biol. Sci. Med. Sci.* **2005**, *60*, 324–333. [PubMed]
4. Han, A.; Bokshan, S.L.; Marcaccio, S.E.; DePasse, J.M.; Daniels, A.H. Diagnostic criteria and clinical outcomes in sarcopenia research: A literature review. *J. Clin. Med.* **2018**, *7*, 70. [CrossRef] [PubMed]
5. Goodpaster, B.H.; Thaete, F.L.; Kelley, D.E. Composition of skeletal muscle evaluated with computed tomography. *Ann. N. Y. Acad. Sci.* **2000**, *904*, 18–24. [CrossRef] [PubMed]
6. Pillen, S.; Tak, R.O.; Zwarts, M.J.; Lammens, M.M.; Verrijp, K.N.; Arts, I.M.; van der Laak, J.A.; Hoogerbruge, P.M.; van Engelen, B.G.; Verrips, A. Skeletal muscle ultrasound: Correlation between fibrous tissue and echo intensity. *Ultrasound Med. Biol.* **2009**, *35*, 443–446. [CrossRef] [PubMed]
7. Pillen, S.; van Dijk, J.P.; Weijers, G.; Raijmann, W.; de Korte, C.L.; Zwarts, M.J. Quantitative gray-scale analysis in skeletal muscle ultrasound: A comparison study of two ultrasound devices. *Muscle Nerve* **2009**, *39*, 781–786. [CrossRef]
8. Arts, I.M.; Pillen, S.; Schelhaas, H.J.; Overeem, S.; Zwarts, M.J. Normal values for quantitative muscle ultrasonography in adults. *Muscle Nerve* **2010**, *41*, 32–41. [CrossRef]
9. Parry, S.M.; El-Ansary, D.; Cartwright, M.S.; Sarwal, A.; Berney, S.; Koopman, R.; Annoni, R.; Puthucheary, Z.; Gordon, I.R.; Morris, P.E.; et al. Ultrasonography in the intensive care setting can be used to detect changes in the quality and quantity of muscle and is related muscle strength and function. *J. Crit. Care* **2015**, *30*, e9–e14. [CrossRef]
10. Puthucheary, Z.A.; Phadke, R.; Rawal, J.; McPhail, M.J.; Sidhu, P.S.; Rowlerson, A.; Moxham, J.; Harridge, S.; Hart, N.; Montgomery, H.E. Qualitative ultrasound in acute critical illness muscle wasting. *Crit. Care Med.* **2015**, *43*, 1603–1611. [CrossRef]

11. Fukumoto, Y.; Ikezoe, T.; Yamada, Y.; Tsukagoshi, R.; Nakamura, M.; Mori, N.; Kimura, M.; Ichihashi, N. Skeletal muscle quality assessed from echo intensity is associated with muscle strength of middle-aged and elderly persons. *Eur. J. Appl. Physiol.* **2012**, *112*, 1519–1525. [CrossRef] [PubMed]
12. Mirón Mombiela, R.; Facal de Castro, F.; Moreno, P.; Borras, C. Ultrasonic echo intensity as a new noninvasive in vivo biomarker of frailty. *J. Am. Geriatr. Soc.* **2017**, *65*, 2685–2690. [CrossRef] [PubMed]
13. Sanchez, B.; Rutkove, S.B. Electrical impedance myography and its applications in neuromuscular disorders. *Neurotherapeutics* **2017**, *14*, 107–118. [CrossRef]
14. Shefner, J.M.; Rutkove, S.B.; Caress, J.B.; Benatar, M.; David, W.S.; Cartwright, M.C.; Macklin, E.A.; Bohoroquez, J.L. Reducing sample size requirements for future ALS clinical trials with a dedicated electrical impedance myography system. *Amyotroph. Lateral Scler. Frontotemporal Degener.* **2018**, *28*, 1–7. [CrossRef] [PubMed]
15. Rutkove, S.B.; Kapur, K.; Zaidman, C.M.; Wu, J.S.; Paternak, A.; Madabusi, L.; Yim, S.; Pacheck, A.; Szelag, H.; Harrington, T.; et al. Electrical impedance myography for assessment of Duchenne muscular dystrophy. *Ann. Neurol.* **2017**, *81*, 622–632. [CrossRef] [PubMed]
16. Zaidman, C.M.; Wang, L.L.; Connolly, A.M.; Florence, J.; Wong, B.L.; Parsons, J.A.; Apkon, S.; Goyal, N.; Williams, E.; Escolar, D.; et al. Electrical impedance myography in Duchenne muscular dystrophy and healthy controls: A multicenter study of reliability and validity. *Muscle Nerve* **2015**, *52*, 592–597. [CrossRef] [PubMed]
17. Ishida, H.; Suehiro, T.; Suzuki, K.; Watanabe, S. Muscle thickness and echo intensity measurements of the rectus femoris muscle of healthy subjects: Intra and interrater reliability of transducer tilt during ultrasound. *J. Bodyw. Mov. Ther.* **2018**, *22*, 657–660. [CrossRef]
18. Toledo, D.O.; Silva, D.C.L.E.; Santos, D.M.D.; Freitas, B.J.; Dib, R.; Cordioli, R.L.; Figueiredo, E.J.A.; Piovacari, S.M.F.; Silva, J.M., Jr. Bedside ultrasound is a practical measurement tool for assessing muscle mass. *Revista Brasileira de Terapia Intensiva* **2017**, *29*, 476–480. [CrossRef]
19. Hadda, V.; Khilnani, G.C.; Kumar, R.; Dhungana, A.; Mittal, S.; Khan, M.A.; Madan, K.; Mohan, A.; Guleria, R. Intra- and inter-observer reliability of quadriceps muscle thickness measured with bedside ultrasonography by critical care physicians. *Indian J. Crit. Care Med.* **2017**, *21*, 448–452. [CrossRef]
20. Thoirs, K.; English, C. Ultrasound measures of muscle thickness: Intra-examiner reliability and influence of body position. *Clin. Physiol. Funct. Imaging* **2009**, *29*, 440–446. [CrossRef]
21. Tillquist, M.; Kutsogiannis, D.J.; Wischmeyer, P.E.; Kummerlen, C.; Leung, R.; Stollery, D.; Karvellas, C.K.; Preiser, J.C.; Bird, N.; Kozar, R.; et al. Bedside ultrasound is a practical and reliable measurement tool for assessing quadriceps muscle layer thickness. *JPEN J. Parenter. Enteral Nutr.* **2014**, *38*, 886–890. [CrossRef] [PubMed]
22. Lopez, P.; Wilhelm, E.N.; Rech, A.; Minozzo, F.; Radaelli, R.; Pinto, R.S. Echo intensity independently predicts functionality in sedentary older men. *Muscle Nerve* **2017**, *55*, 9–15. [CrossRef] [PubMed]
23. Rech, A.; Radaelli, R.; Goltz, F.R.; da Rosa, L.H.; Schneider, C.D.; Pinto, R.S. Echo intensity is negatively associated with functional capacity in older women. *Age* **2014**, *36*, 9708. [CrossRef]
24. Aaron, R.; Esper, G.J.; Shiffman, C.A.; Bradonjic, K.; Lee, K.S.; Rutkove, S.B. Effects of age on muscle as measured by electrical impedance myography. *Physiol. Meas.* **2006**, *27*, 953–959. [CrossRef]
25. Kortman, H.G.; Wilder, S.C.; Geisbush, T.R.; Narayanaswami, P.; Rutkove, S.B. Age- and gender-associated differences in electrical impedance values of skeletal muscle. *Physiol. Meas.* **2013**, *34*, 1611–1622. [CrossRef]
26. McLester, C.N.; Dewitt, A.D.; Rooks, R.; McLester, J.R. An investigation of the accuracy and reliability of body composition assessed with a handheld electrical impedance myography device. *Eur. J. Sport Sci.* **2018**, *18*, 763–771. [CrossRef]
27. Geisbush, T.R.; Visyak, N.; Madabusi, L.; Rutkove, S.B.; Darras, B.T. Inter-session reliability of electrical impedance myography in children in a clinical trial setting. *Clin. Neurophysiol.* **2015**, *126*, 1790–1796. [CrossRef] [PubMed]
28. O'Brien, T.G.; Cazares Gonzalez, M.L.; Ghosh, P.S.; Mandrekar, J.; Boon, A.J. Reliability of a novel ultrasound system for gray-scale analysis of muscle. *Muscle Nerve* **2017**, *56*, 408–412. [CrossRef]

© 2018 by the authors. Licensee MDPI, Basel, Switzerland. This article is an open access article distributed under the terms and conditions of the Creative Commons Attribution (CC BY) license (http://creativecommons.org/licenses/by/4.0/).

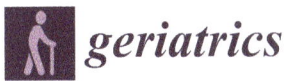

Communication

The Clinical Frailty Scale: Do Staff Agree?

Rebekah L. Young [1,*] and David G. Smithard [2,3]

1. Newham University Hospital, Bart's Health NHS Trust, London E13 8SL, UK
2. Queen Elizabeth Hospital, Lewisham and Greenwich NHS Trust, London SE18 4QH, UK; david.smithard@nhs.net
3. Department of Sports Science, University of Greenwich, London SE10 9BD, UK
* Correspondence: rebekah.young5@nhs.net

Received: 18 May 2020; Accepted: 16 June 2020; Published: 25 June 2020

Abstract: The term frailty is being increasingly used by clinicians, however there is no strict consensus on the best screening method. The expectation in England is that all older patients should have the Clinical Frailty Scale (CFS) completed on admission. This will frequently rely on junior medical staff and nurses, raising the question as to whether there is consistency. We asked 124 members of a multidisciplinary team (consultants, junior doctors, nurses, and allied health professionals; physiotherapists, occupational therapists, dietitians, speech and language therapists) to complete the CFS for seven case scenarios. The majority of the participants, 91/124 (72%), were trainee medical staff, 16 were senior medical staff, 12 were allied health professions, and 6 were nurses. There was broad agreement both between the professions and within the professions, with median CFS scores varying by a maximum of only one point, except in case scenario G, where there was a two-point difference between the most junior trainees (FY1) and the nursing staff. No difference (using the Mann–Whitney U test) was found between the different staff groups, with the median scores and range of scores being similar. This study has confirmed there is agreement between different staff members when calculating the CFS with no specific preceding training.

Keywords: frailty; clinical frailty score

1. Introduction

Frailty can be described as a clinical state in which the ability of older people to cope with every-day or acute stressors is compromised by increased vulnerability due to age-associated declines in physiological reserve and function across multiple organ systems [1]. It is estimated that around 10% of people aged over 65 years are frail, which increases to 25–50% of those aged over 85 [2]. Frailty can also be used to describe certain physical changes, such as muscle wasting and weakness, leading to reduced walking ability. The identification of these patients allows us to start a care pathway to address the issues contributing to frailty and avoid adverse outcomes.

All older people admitted to hospital should undergo a comprehensive geriatric assessment (CGA). It is recommended that this should commence on the day of admission [3]. An assessment of frailty is one component of the CGA, and similarly should be completed at the earliest opportunity. Assessments of frailty (frailty scales) are numerous [4] and rely on the recall of information, either by the patient or carer. The term frailty is being increasingly used by clinicians, however there is no strict consensus on the most appropriate screening scale [4].

The Clinical Frailty Scale, first described by Rockwood et al. in 2005 [5], is a nine-point scale where the assessor makes a judgement about the degree of a person's frailty based upon clinical assessment and has been adopted by the Acute Frailty Network in the UK. The advantage the CFS has over other scales is that it offers a pictorial representation with a small description and is quick and simple to administer.

As the various frailty scores measure slightly different things, it is possible to score as severely frail on one and moderately frail on another. It is therefore important that the same scale is used throughout any one service.

The expectation in England is that all older patients should have the Clinical Frailty Scale completed at the time of admission or soon after [6]. This will frequently rely on the junior trainee medical staff and nurses. This raises the question as to whether there is consistency in completing the assessments.

2. Methodology

The participants (consultants, junior doctors, nurses, and allied health professionals; physiotherapists, occupational therapists, dietitians, speech and language therapists) were approached on the ward and at time of clinical education sessions/conferences. A total of 124 people agreed to take part (Table 1). They were provided with seven clinical case scenarios (Table 2) based on actual clinical scenarios and asked to provide a frailty score by referring to the Clinical Frailty Scale (1–9) (Figure 1). The results were completed anonymously; participants were requested to provide their profession and grade where appropriate. The participants had no or limited experience using the CFS, nor was any training provided on how to use it. The nurses and allied health professionals were of varying levels of qualification, from newly qualified to senior staff.

Clinical Frailty Scale*

1 Very Fit – People who are robust, active, energetic and motivated. These people commonly exercise regularly. They are among the fittest for their age.

2 Well – People who have **no active disease symptoms** but are less fit than category 1. Often, they exercise or are very **active occasionally**, e.g. seasonally.

3 Managing Well – People whose **medical problems are well controlled,** but are **not regularly active** beyond routine walking.

4 Vulnerable – While **not dependent** on others for daily help, often **symptoms limit activities**. A common complaint is being "slowed up", and/or being tired during the day.

5 Mildly Frail – These people often have **more evident slowing**, and need help in **high order IADLs** (finances, transportation, heavy housework, medications). Typically, mild frailty progressively impairs shopping and walking outside alone, meal preparation and housework.

6 Moderately Frail – People need help with **all outside activities** and with **keeping house**. Inside, they often have problems with stairs and need **help with bathing** and might need minimal assistance (cuing, standby) with dressing.

7 Severely Frail – **Completely dependent for personal care**, from whatever cause (physical or cognitive). Even so, they seem stable and not at high risk of dying (within ~ 6 months).

8 Very Severely Frail – Completely dependent, approaching the end of life. Typically, they could not recover even from a minor illness.

9. Terminally Ill – Approaching the end of life. This category applies to people with **a life expectancy <6 months**, who are **not otherwise evidently frail**.

Scoring frailty in people with dementia

The degree of frailty corresponds to the degree of dementia. Common **symptoms in mild dementia** include forgetting the details of a recent event, though still remembering the event itself, repeating the same question/story and social withdrawal.

In **moderate dementia**, recent memory is very impaired, even though they seemingly can remember their past life events well. They can do personal care with prompting.

In **severe dementia**, they cannot do personal care without help.

* 1. Canadian Study on Health & Aging, Revised 2008.
2. K. Rockwood et al. A global clinical measure of fitness and frailty in elderly people. CMAJ 2005;173:489-495.

© 2007-2009 Version 1.2. All rights reserved. Geriatric Medicine Research, Dalhousie University, Halifax, Canada. Permission granted to copy for research and educational purposes only.

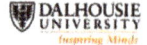

Figure 1. The Clinical Frailty Scale (CFS) [5].

Table 1. Description of staff groups and previous experience with the CFS.

Staff Grade	Years Qualified	Experience with CFS
FY1	Immediately post qualification	None
SHO	Second year post training (may be longer depending on the individual)	None
Registrar	Min 4 years after undergraduate training	A few may have used the CFS
Consultant	At least nine years post graduate training	Depending on Specialty. Geriatricians would have experience other specialties not
Nursing/ AHP	Mixed 1–20	No exposure to CFS

Table 2. Clinical case scenarios.

	Case History
A.	84-year-old male. Admitted with a fall. Lives alone. Independent washing and dressing. Uses a walking stick in the house, housebound. Problems with urinary incontinence and wears pads. Has a BD care package when son away.
B.	81-year-old female. Walks with a Zimmer frame. Single level living. Undertakes a strip wash. Needs help with dressing, cooking, cleaning, shopping. Housebound. Carers 4 times a day. Unable to manage finances.
C.	91-year-old male. Independent with transfers from bed to chair but help otherwise to transfer chair to commode. Walks with a Zimmer frame but needs assistance. Help with personal activities of daily living (ADLs) (washing, dressing, shaving). Continence is an issue. Short term memory problems. Housebound. Unable to manage finances.
D.	74-year-old female. Working in an office, independent and self-caring. Drives a car. No care issues.
E.	89-year-old female. Walks with a stick and uses a 4-wheel shopper. Beginning to struggle with transfers (out of chair, off toilet) and lower half dressing. No package of care.
F.	84-year-old female. Recurrent falls and troubles with medication. Housebound, carers three times a day. Continent. Help with cooking, shopping and dressing. Requires help with medication. Cannot manage finances.
G.	82-year-old female. Falls, dementia. Independently mobile. Out shopping. Walks with a stick. Independent with personal and extended ADLS.

3. Results

The majority of participants—91/124 (72%)—were trainee medical staff, 16 were senior medical staff, 12 were allied health professions, and 6 were nurses (Figure 2).

There was broad agreement both between the professions and within the professions, with median CFS scores varying by a maximum of only one point, except in case scenario G, where there was a two-point difference between the most junior trainees (FY1) and the nursing staff (Figure 3). No difference (using multiple Mann–Whitney U) was found between different staff groups (basis between any two groups), with the median scores and range of scores all being very similar.

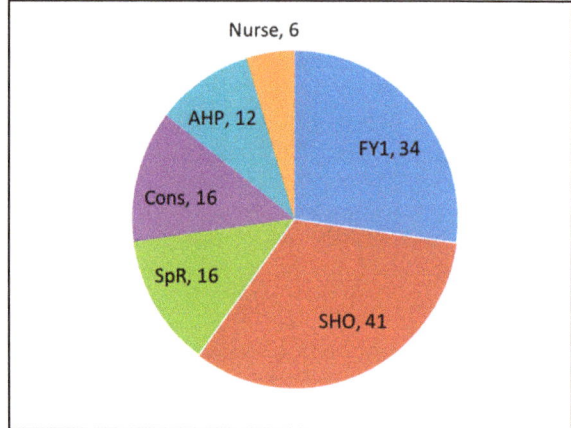

Figure 2. Distribution of staff completing the study.

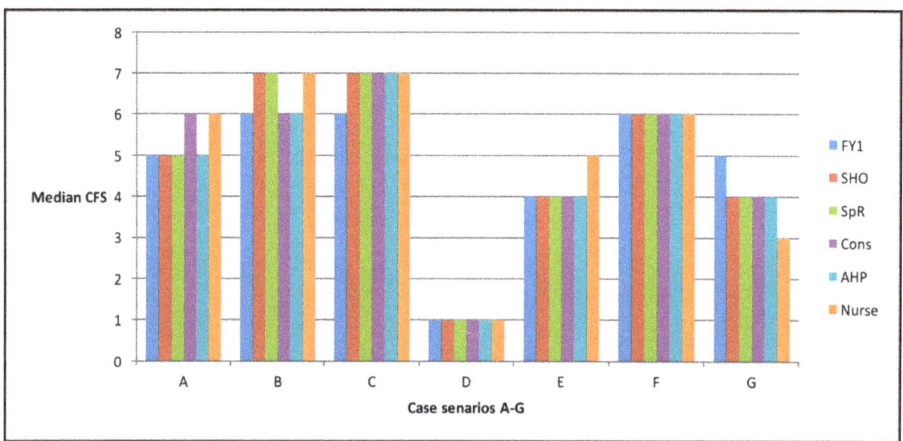

Figure 3. Chart to show the median CFS score calculated for each case scenario, divided by the member of the multidisciplinary team completing the score.

4. Discussion

The severity of prior frailty at the time of admission is a prognostic indicator of outcome (length of stay, institutionalisation, and mortality) from acute medical and surgical illness [7–10]. Holistic medical management uses information from many sources, one of which is a frailty scale. For any tool to be adopted into clinical practice, it needs to be simple and quick to use. The CFS meets both criteria (Figure 1) and is used widely used in many geriatric services in England; however, the CFS, like any other assessment tool, needs to be consistent in identifying and grading frailty between clinical staff and between clinical services.

In a study conducted by a university-associated tertiary hospital in Melbourne, Australia, all patients aged 65 and over admitted to the general medical unit during August and September 2013 had their baseline CFS score documented by a member of the treating medical team [11]. Despite the lack of prior training for medical staff on the use of the CFS, increasing frailty was correlated with functional decline and mortality, supporting the validity of the CFS as a frailty screening tool for clinicians. This study, however, did not compare the scores between staff groups.

In a retrospective note review by a medical student, a CFS was completed and then compared to one completed by a nurse specialist during a comprehensive geriatric assessment. The agreement between the two assessments, using Cohen's Kappa, was 0.63 [12]. An ICU-based study compared medical students with ICU doctors completing the CFS during patients' stays and again found an agreement of 0.64 [13]. Rolfson et al. found a good interrater reliability with the Edmonton Frailty Scale completed by Geriatric specialist nurses [14].

In this study, the largest disagreement was with case scenario G, where there was a two-point difference between the most junior trainees (FY1) and the nursing staff. This could be explained by the fact the patient was independent with activities of daily living, but also suffering from falls, indicating that she may need more help. Overall, there was broad agreement, and therefore the CFS can be documented on patient admission and we can be reassured of the score's consistency, despite it being used by different staff groups. The routine identification of frailty is good practice, as the identification of these patients allows us to start a care pathway to address the issues contributing to frailty and avoid adverse outcomes.

5. Conclusions

This study has confirmed that there is agreement between different staff members when conducting the CFS with no specific preceding training.

Author Contributions: Both authors contributed to the design and implementation of the research, D.G.S. performed data analysis, and both authors assisted in writing the manuscript. All authors have read and agreed to the published version of the manuscript.

Funding: This research received no external funding.

Conflicts of Interest: There are no conflicts of interest.

References

1. WHO Clinical Consortium on Healthy Ageing: Topic Focus: Frailty and Intrinsic Capacity: Report of Consortium Meeting, 2016 in Geneva, Switzerland. Available online: https://www.who.int/ageing/health-systems/first-CCHA-meeting-report.pdf?ua=1 (accessed on 24 June 2020).
2. Romero-Ortuno, R.; O'Shea, D. Fitness and frailty: opposite ends of a challenging continuum! Will the end of age discrimination make frailty assessments an imperative? *Age Ageing* **2013**, *42*, 279–280. [CrossRef] [PubMed]
3. British Geriatrics Society, Fit for frailty guideline. Available online: https://www.bgs.org.uk/sites/default/files/content/resources/files/2018-05-23/fff_full.pdf (accessed on 24 June 2020).
4. Wou, F.; Gladman, J.; Bradshaw, L.; Franklin, M.; Edmans, J.; Conroy, S. The predictive properties of frailty-rating scales in the acute medical unit. *Eur. Geriatr. Med.* **2013**, *4*, S74. [CrossRef]
5. Rockwood, K.; Song, X.; Macknight, C.; Bergman, H.; Hogan, D.B.; McDowell, I.; Mitnitski, A. A global clinical measure of fitness and frailty in elderly people. *Can. Med Assoc. J.* **2005**, *173*, 489–495. [CrossRef] [PubMed]
6. Specialised Clinical Frailty Network, the Clinical Frailty Scale. Available online: https://www.scfn.org.uk/clinical-frailty-scale (accessed on 24 June 2020).
7. Darvall, J.N.; Bellomo, R.; Paul, E.; Subramaniam, A.; Santamaria, J.D.; Bagshaw, S.M.; Rai, S.; E Hubbard, R.; Pilcher, D. Frailty in very old critically ill patients in Australia and New Zealand: a population-based cohort study. *Med J. Aust.* **2019**, *211*, 318–323. [CrossRef] [PubMed]
8. O'Caoimh, R.; Costello, M.; Small, C.; Spooner, L.; Flannery, A.; O'Reilly, L.; Heffernan, L.; Mannion, E.; Maughan, A.; Joyce, A.; et al. Comparison of Frailty Screening Instruments in the Emergency Department. *Int. J. Environ. Res. Public Heal.* **2019**, *16*, 3626. [CrossRef] [PubMed]
9. Kahlon, S.; Pederson, J.; Majumdar, S.R.; Belga, S.; Lau, D.; Fradette, M.; Boyko, D.; Bakal, J.A.; Johnston, C.; Padwal, R.; et al. Association between frailty and 30-day outcomes after discharge from hospital. *Can. Med Assoc. J.* **2015**, *187*, 799–804. [CrossRef] [PubMed]

10. Patel, K.V.; Brennan, K.L.; Brennan, M.L.; Jupiter, D.C.; Shar, A.; Davis, M.L. Association of a Modified Frailty Index With Mortality After Femoral Neck Fracture in Patients Aged 60 Years and Older. *Clin. Orthop. Relat. Res.* **2013**, *472*, 1010–1017. [CrossRef] [PubMed]
11. Gregorevic, K.J.; E Hubbard, R.; Lim, W.K.; Katz, B. The clinical frailty scale predicts functional decline and mortality when used by junior medical staff: a prospective cohort study. *BMC Geriatr.* **2016**, *16*, 117. [CrossRef] [PubMed]
12. Davies, J.; Whitlock, J.; Gutmanis, I.; Kane, S.-L. Inter-Rater Reliability of the Retrospectively Assigned Clinical Frailty Scale Score in a Geriatric Outreach Population. *Can. Geriatr. J.* **2018**, *21*, 1–5. [CrossRef] [PubMed]
13. Pugh, R.; Ellison, A.; Pye, K.; Subbe, C.P.; Thorpe, C.M.; Lone, N.; Clegg, A. Feasibility and reliability of frailty assessment in the critically ill: a systematic review. *Crit. Care* **2018**, *22*, 49. [CrossRef] [PubMed]
14. Rolfson, D.B.; Majumdar, S.R.; Tsuyuki, R.T.; Tahir, A.; Rockwood, K. Validity and reliability of the Edmonton frailty score. *Age and Ageing* **2006**, *35*, 526–529. [CrossRef] [PubMed]

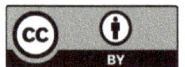

© 2020 by the authors. Licensee MDPI, Basel, Switzerland. This article is an open access article distributed under the terms and conditions of the Creative Commons Attribution (CC BY) license (http://creativecommons.org/licenses/by/4.0/).

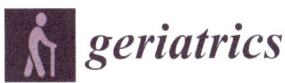

Article

The Convergent Validity of the electronic Frailty Index (eFI) with the Clinical Frailty Scale (CFS)

Antoinette Broad [1], Ben Carter [2], Sara Mckelvie [3,4] and Jonathan Hewitt [5,*]

[1] Community Services, Oxford Health NHS Foundation Trust, Oxford OX3 7JX, UK; antoinette.broad@oxfordhealth.nhs.uk
[2] Department of Biostatistics and Health Informatics, Institute of Psychiatry, Psychology & Neuroscience, King's College London, London SE5 8AF, UK; ben.carter@kcl.ac.uk
[3] Emergency Medical Unit, Oxford Health NHS Foundation Trust, Oxford OX3 7JX, UK; sara.mckelvie@oxfordhealth.nhs.uk or S.Mckelvie@soton.ac.uk
[4] Primary Care Research Group, Faculty of Medicine, University of Southampton, Southampton SO17 1BJ, UK
[5] Division of Population Medicine, Cardiff University, Penarth CF64 2XX, UK
* Correspondence: hewittj2@cardiff.ac.uk

Received: 6 September 2020; Accepted: 28 September 2020; Published: 9 November 2020

Abstract: Background: Different scales are being used to measure frailty. This study examined the convergent validity of the electronic Frailty Index (eFI) with the Clinical Frailty Scale (CFS). **Method:** The cross-sectional study recruited patients from three regional community nursing teams in the South East of England. The CFS was rated at recruitment, and the eFI was extracted from electronic health records (EHRs). A McNemar test of paired data was used to compare discordant pairs between the eFI and the CFS, and an exact McNemar Odds Ratio (OR) was calculated. **Findings:** Of 265 eligible patients consented, 150 (57%) were female, with a mean age of 85.6 years (SD = 7.8), and 78% were 80 years and older. Using the CFS, 68% were estimated to be moderate to severely frail, compared to 91% using the eFI. The eFI recorded a greater degree of frailty than the CFS (OR = 5.43, 95%CI 3.05 to 10.40; $p < 0.001$). This increased to 7.8 times more likely in men, and 9.5 times in those aged over 80 years. **Conclusions:** This study found that the eFI overestimates the frailty status of community dwelling older people. Overestimating frailty may impact on the demand of resources required for further management and treatment of those identified as being frail.

Keywords: clinical Frailty Scale; electronic Frailty Index; community

1. Introduction

Frailty has been defined as a state of vulnerability to adverse outcomes, as a consequence of cumulative decline in physiological systems and homeostatic reserve over the course of an individual's lifetime [1]. Frailty is a distinct syndrome independent of disease [2].

With populations worldwide ageing rapidly frailty is high on everyone's agenda, although the concept is well recognised, an international consensus to define frailty has yet to be reached [3]. In the absence of such a gold standard, many tools have been developed [4]. A standard measurement tool would provide a consistent recognition of frailty [5].

Due to age-related changes, frailty is diagnosed more often in older people [5]. Early identification of frailty can decrease the burden of disease, maintain independence longer and improve quality of life [6]. In response to this increasing evidence, NHS England published a new NHS long term plan [7] which calls for more proactive approaches to targeting interventions appropriately whilst contractually obliging General Practitioners (GPs) to identify patients over the age of 65 with moderate to severe frailty [8]. One frailty measure, the electronic Frailty Index (eFI) can be calculated by GPs using existing software and has become the GPs' preferred frailty tool [9]. The Clinical Frailty Scale (CFS) is another validated measure of frailty based on clinical presentation. It is commonly used in clinical practice to diagnose frailty due to its simplicity [10]. It is essential that frailty is reproducible across different instruments used to identify it (convergent validity).

The study aimed to examine the convergent validity of the electronic Frailty Index (eFI) [11] with the 9- point Clinical Frailty Scale (CFS) [12] on community dwelling older people admitted onto a community nursing caseload.

2. Materials and Methods

2.1. Study Design

An observational design across three sites in the UK. The study was conducted in December 2018. As data used were collected as part of routine care, the study was deemed a service evaluation and was registered locally.

2.2. Participants

Community dwelling people (65 years or over) accepted on to three separate community nursing caseloads during one week in December 2018 were eligible to participate. Selected community nursing caseloads were determined by the following factors: geographical area, number of GP practices and location; city, town or village. Participants excluded from the study were those aged below 65 years.

2.3. Measures

The eFI is a cumulative deficit model that calculates frailty by retrieving patient information recorded from the electronic health record (EHR) [11]. It includes 36 deficit variables derived from diseases, symptoms and clinical signs recorded on the EHR. It can be calculated automatically on the EHR without the oversight of a clinician. Supplementary Table S1 shows the 36 deficits. It includes physical limitations including requirement of care, activity, mobility and transfer problems. It divides the total number of deficits present by the total possible creating a score between 0-1. The deficits each have a binary score of 1 if present and 0 when absent. eFI = Sum of deficits/36 (total number of deficits). The score is categorised accordingly into levels of severity, 0–0.12 = fit; >0.12–0.24 = mild frailty; >0.24–0.36 = moderate frailty and above 0.36 = severely frail [11].

The nine category Clinical Frailty Scale (CFS), is a validated measure of frailty based on clinical presentation. The assessor judges the level of frailty based on clinical findings and includes physical disability, cognition and co morbidity. It scores between one (very fit) to nine (terminally ill with a life expectancy of <6 months) [12]. Each point on the scale corresponds with a picture and written description to assist the clinician to grade the frailty score, a score = or >5 is frail [13]. Supplementary Figure S1 demonstrates the CFS.

2.4. Scoring Frailty

2.4.1. eFI

Trained senior community nurses extracted the participants personal demographic data from community nursing teams' EHR then accessed the participants eFI scores from the GP practice EHR.

2.4.2. CFS

An assessment of frailty using the CFS was completed in the participants' home during routine visits by community nurses within one week of their eFI screening. Training on how to complete the CFS was delivered by the study team. Nurses using the CFS were blinded to the recorded eFI score and classification. Participants were categorised as fit/mild or moderate/severely frail based on their reported scores.

The CFS and eFI were both dichotomised into two comparable scores of fit/mildly frail (CFS very fit, to mildly frail; eFI fit, to mildly frail), and moderately/severely frail (CFS moderately frail to terminally frail; eFI moderate to severely frail).

2.5. Statistical Analysis

Descriptive statistics were used to describe the population demographics and the distribution of frailty. Both the eFI and CFS were categorised into fit/mild, and moderate/severe. Categorisation of CFS followed the literature and 1–5 was compared to CFS 6–9, [14,15]; eFI was less common reported, and we mapped across a consistent threshold for this tool.

The McNemar test was used to test the association between the rating of the two frailty instruments: the eFI and the CFS [16]. The odds ratio (OR) and 95% confidence interval of over estimating frailty was calculated using the discordant pairs (e.g., comparing those more frail in the eFI (but not the CFS), was compared with those more frail in the CFS (but not the eFI)).

A subgroup analysis included patients aged over 80 years, as well as by gender. All analyses were carried out using Stata version 15.0.

3. Results

A total of 365 patients were recorded on the caseload, of which 327 met the eligibility criteria, 62 were removed due to incomplete data. Of those included, 150 (57%) were female, with a mean age of 85.6 years (SD = 7.8), and 78% were 80 years and older. Frailty prevalence estimates of moderate/severe were 91% (eFI), and 68% (CFS). (Table 1). There was a higher proportion of female patients in the moderate/severely frail group, but similar proportions of men and women in the fit/mildly frail group. Association between the frailty instruments was assessed by discordant pair analysis (Table 2).

Table 1. Demographic characteristics of the study population.

Category of Frailty	eFI		CFS	
	Fit/Mild	Moderate/Severe	Fit/Mild	Moderate/Severe
Total patients	23 (9%)	242 (91%)	85 (32%)	180 (68%)
Age (mean)	80.7	86	84.8	85.95
Male	10 (43%)	105 (43%)	43 (51%)	72 (40%)
Female	13 (57%)	137 (57%)	42 (49%)	108 (60%)

Table 2. Association between the electronic Frailty Index (eFI) and the Clinical Frailty Scale (CFS).

		CFS		
	Category of frailty	Fit to Mild	Moderate to Severe	Total
eFI	Fit to Mild	9	14	23
	Moderate to severe	76	166	242
	Total	85	180	265

Looking at the discordant pairs there were 76 patients seen by a clinician and found to have fit/mild frailty via the CFS but recorded moderate/severe frailty using the eFI, and inversely 14 patients scored moderate/severe with the CFS but as fit/mildly frail with the eFI. There was very strong evidence of an association of difference in the rate of discordant pairs ($p < 0.001$), and indication that the eFI is recorded with a greater degree of frailty. A patient being scored as more severely frail using the eFI compared to the CFS exhibited an OR = 5.43, (95%CI 3.05 to 10.40; $p < 0.001$).

Subgroup analysis estimated that this over scoring was more extreme in patients who were over 80 years old ($p < 0.001$), and in men ($p < 0.001$) (Table 3).

Table 3. Subgroup of electronic Frailty Index (eFI) and the Clinical Frailty Scale (CFS) scores by age.

≤80 years	CFS		
eFI	Mild/fit	Moderate/severe	Total
Mild/fit	4 (a)	8 (b)	12 (a + b)
Moderate/severe	19 (c)	39 (d)	58 (c + d)
total	23 (a + c)	47 (b + d)	70
>80 years	CFS		
eFI	Mild/fit	Moderate/severe	Total
Mild/fit	5 (a)	6 (b)	11 (a + b)
Moderate/severe	57 (c)	127 (d)	184 (c + d)
total	62 (a + c)	133 (b + d)	195

4. Discussion

This study found no evidence of convergent validity and the findings suggest that the eFI overestimates frailty among community dwelling older people. This overestimation increased for people greater than 80 years and for men. These findings conflict with recent studies that support the convergent validity of the two instruments [11,17] and endorse the eFI as a valid case finding tool to identify moderate/severely frail patients who may benefit from targeted interventions [11,18,19].

One explanation for the heterogeneity between scores might be that the two frailty instruments are underpinned by two very different theoretical frameworks. The CFS has been used widely (most recently during the COVID-19 pandemic) and has clinical judgement and has good face validity, it requires clinicians to undertake assessments of their patients' comorbidities in real time [20]. Time to complete the CFS assessment and staff training are two main factors that limit the use of the CFS in practice [21]. In contrast the eFI is quick and requires minimal resources to complete; an accumulative deficit tool can be generated automatically on the GP system [11]. Utilising GP records for collecting patient data to assess frailty has been hailed as the gold standard [22]. The eFI is reliant upon clinicians applying clinical judgement and recording patient data accurately, and poor recording on the EHR can lead to absences of deficits or deficits can remain, even for temporary conditions [18]. Deficits no longer relevant to the patient's current health state can lead to the eFI score being a biased estimate, potentially resulting in the reporting of the patient's poorest estimate of frailty.

A second explanation for the divergent scores may be due to the population as housebound populations are often frail [23] so the findings from this study may not be comparable to the other studies that targeted total populations, their findings reported much lower levels of frailty [11]. Participants in the other studies that supported the convergent validity of the eFI and CFS were also less frail and younger than this study population [11,17]. This could offer an explanation as to why the scores were so different in that the eFI exhibited the worst status of the patient's frailty and the convergent validity of the eFI and CFS may only be true for a younger, fit/mildly frail population. This study sample size and targeted population may limit the generalisability of the study findings.

5. Conclusions

The eFI has been recommended as a screening tool for frailty in primary care. This study suggests that the CFS offers current utility and the eFI overestimates the degree of frailty among housebound, older people, so use of the eFI may deplete health resources by directing services to people who do not require them. Thus, CFS should be preferred over the eFI. We recommend replicating this study on a larger scale to explore the above findings in more detail and to investigate the eFI as a case finding tool.

By having a greater understanding of frailty, clinicians can identify those at greatest risk of adverse health outcomes. Assessing frailty in older people over 65 years is now mandated in primary care in

England [8]. The eFI is a popular choice due to its accessibility and ease of use but it may overestimate a patient's true frailty status.

Supplementary Materials: The following are available online at http://www.mdpi.com/2308-3417/5/4/88/s1, Figure S1: Clinical Frailty Scale (CFS), Table S1: eFI list of 36 health deficits.

Author Contributions: Conceptualisation, A.B., J.H. and S.M.; methodology, A.B., J.H.; software, A.B., B.C.; validation, A.B., J.H., B.C. and S.M.; formal analysis, A.B., B.C., J.H.; investigation, A.B.; resources, A.B.; data curation; A.B., B.C., J.H.; writing—original draft preparation, A.B.; writing—review and editing, J.H., B.C. and S.M.; supervision, J.H.; project administration, A.B. All authors have read and agreed to the published version of the manuscript.

Funding: This research received no external funding.

Conflicts of Interest: The authors declare no conflict of interest.

References

1. Clegg, A.; Rogers, L.; Young, J. Diagnostic test accuracy of simple instruments for identifying frailty in community-dwelling older people: A systematic review. *Age Ageing* **2014**, *44*, 148–152. [CrossRef] [PubMed]
2. Chen, C.Y.; Gan, P.; How, C.H. Approach to frailty in the elderly in primary care and the community. *Singap. Med. J.* **2018**, *59*, 240–245. [CrossRef] [PubMed]
3. John, P.D.S.; McClement, S.S.; Swift, A.U.; Tate, R.B. Older Men's Definitions of Frailty—The Manitoba Follow-up Study. *Can. J. Aging* **2018**, *38*, 13–20. [CrossRef] [PubMed]
4. Gilardi, F.; Capanna, A.; Ferraro, M.; Scarcella, P.; Marazzi, M.C.; Palombi, L.; Liotta, G. Frailty screening and assessment tools: A review of characteristics and use in Public Health. *Ann. Ig.* **2018**, *30*, 128–139. [PubMed]
5. Dent, E.; Kowal, P.; Hoogendijk, E.O. Frailty measurement in research and clinical practice: A review. *Eur. J. Intern. Med.* **2016**, *31*, 3–10. [CrossRef] [PubMed]
6. British Geriatric Society (BGS). Comprehensive Geriatric Assessment Toolkit for Primary Care Practitioners (online). 2019. Available online: https://www.bgs.org.uk/resources/resource-series/comprehensive-geriatric-assessment-toolkit-for-primary-care-practitioners (accessed on 10 July 2020).
7. NHS England. NHS Long Term Plan (online). 2019. Available online: https://www.longtermplan.nhs.uk/online-version/ (accessed on 4 July 2020).
8. NHS England. Supporting Routine Frailty Identification and Frailty through the GP Contract 2017/2018 (online). 2019. Available online: https://www.england.nhs.uk/publication/supporting-routine-frailty-identification-and-frailty-through-the-gp-contract-20172018/ (accessed on 7 July 2020).
9. Stow, D.; Matthews, F.E.; Barclay, S.; Iliffe, S.; Clegg, A.; De Biase, S.; Robinson, L.; Hanratty, B. Evaluating frailty scores to predict mortality in older adults using data from population based electronic health records: Case control study. *Age Ageing* **2018**, *47*, 564–569. [CrossRef] [PubMed]
10. Long, S.; Jelley, B.; Martin, R.; Suter-Jones, V.E. Underestimation of frailty using the 7-point Clinical Frailty Scale: An evaluation of geriatric registrar scoring accuracy. *Age Ageing* **2018**, *47*, ii25–ii39. [CrossRef]
11. Clegg, A.P.; Bates, C.; Young, J.; Ryan, R.; Nichols, L.; Teale, E.A.; Mohammed, M.A.; Parry, J.; Marshall, T. Development and validation of an electronic frailty index using routine primary care electronic health record data. *Age Ageing* **2016**, *45*, 353–360. [CrossRef] [PubMed]
12. Rockwood, K.; Song, X.; Macknight, C.; Bergman, H.; Hogan, D.; McDowell, I.; Mitnitski, A. A global clinical measure of fitness and frailty in elderly people. *Can. Med Assoc. J.* **2005**, *173*, 489–495. [CrossRef] [PubMed]
13. Ozsurekci, C.; Balcı, C.; Kızılarslanoğlu, M.C.; Çalışkan, H.; Doğrul, R.T.; Ayçiçek, G. Şengül; Sümer, F.; Karabulut, E.; Yavuz, B.B.; Cankurtaran, M.; et al. An important problem in an aging country: Identifying the frailty via 9 Point Clinical Frailty Scale. *Acta Clin. Belg.* **2019**, *75*, 200–204. [CrossRef] [PubMed]
14. Owen, R.K.; Conroy, S.P.; Taub, N.; Jones, W.; Bryden, D.; Pareek, M.; Faull, C.; Abrams, K.R.; Davis, D.; Banerjee, J. OUP accepted manuscript. *Age Ageing* **2020**. [CrossRef]
15. Aw, D.; Woodrow, L.; Ogliari, G.; Harwood, R. Association of frailty with mortality in older inpatients with Covid-19: A cohort study. *Age Ageing* **2020**. [CrossRef] [PubMed]
16. Upton, G.J.; Cook, I. *A Dictionary of Statistics*; Oxford University Press: Oxford, UK, 2006.
17. Brundle, C.; Heaven, A.; Brown, L.; Teale, E.; Young, J.; West, R.; Clegg, A. Convergent validity of the electronic frailty index. *Age Ageing* **2018**, *48*, 152–156. [CrossRef] [PubMed]

18. Abbasi, M.; Khera, S.; Dabravolskaj, J.; Vandermeer, B.; Theou, O.; Rolfson, D.; Clegg, A. A cross-sectional study examining convergent validity of a frailty index based on electronic medical records in a Canadian primary care program. *BMC Geriatr.* **2019**, *19*, 109.
19. Lansbury, L.N.; Roberts, H.C.; Clift, E.; Herklots, A.; Robinson, N.; Sayer, A.A. Use of the electronic Frailty Index to identify vulnerable patients: A pilot study in primary care. *Br. J. Gen. Pr.* **2017**, *67*, e751–e756. [CrossRef] [PubMed]
20. Hewitt, J.; Carter, B.; Vilches-Moraga, A.; Quinn, T.J.; Braude, P.; Verduri, A.; Pearce, L.; Stechman, M.; Short, R.; Price, A.; et al. The effect of frailty on survival in patients with COVID-19 (COPE): A multicentre, European, observational cohort study. *Lancet Public Health* **2020**, *5*, e444–e451. [CrossRef]
21. Elliott, A.; Phelps, K.; Regen, E.; Conroy, S.P. Identifying frailty in the Emergency Department—Feasibility study. *Age Ageing* **2017**, *46*, 840–845. [CrossRef] [PubMed]
22. Hale, M.D.; Santorelli, G.; Brundle, C.; Clegg, A. A cross-sectional study assessing agreement between self-reported and general practice-recorded health conditions among community dwelling older adults. *Age Ageing* **2019**, *49*, 135–140. [CrossRef] [PubMed]
23. Qiu, W.; Dean, M.; Liu, T.; George, L.; Gann, M.; Cohen, J.; Bruce, M.L. Physical and mental health of homebound older adults: An overlooked population. *J. Am. Geriatr. Soc.* **2010**, *58*, 2423–2428. [CrossRef] [PubMed]

Publisher's Note: MDPI stays neutral with regard to jurisdictional claims in published maps and institutional affiliations.

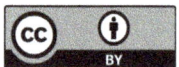

© 2020 by the authors. Licensee MDPI, Basel, Switzerland. This article is an open access article distributed under the terms and conditions of the Creative Commons Attribution (CC BY) license (http://creativecommons.org/licenses/by/4.0/).

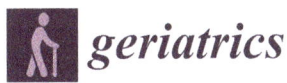

Article

Geriatric Resource Teams: Equipping Primary Care Practices to Meet the Complex Care Needs of Older Adults

Gwendolen Buhr [1,*], Carrissa Dixon [2], Jan Dillard [3,4], Elissa Nickolopoulos [3,4], Lynn Bowlby [3], Holly Canupp [3,5], Loretta Matters [6], Thomas Konrad [7], Laura Previll [1,8], Mitchell Heflin [1,8] and Eleanor McConnell [1,6,8]

1. Duke Center for the Study of Aging and Human Development, Durham, NC 27710, USA; laura.previll@duke.edu (L.P.); mitchell.heflin@duke.edu (M.H.); eleanor.mcconnell@duke.edu (E.M.)
2. Duke Office of Clinical Research, Durham, NC 27710, USA; carrissa.dixon@duke.edu
3. Duke Outpatient Clinic, Durham, NC 27704, USA; janice.dillard@duke.edu (J.D.); elissa.rumer@duke.edu (E.N.); lynn.bowlby@duke.edu (L.B.); holly.causey@duke.edu (H.C.)
4. Department of Case Management and Clinical Social Work, Duke University Medical Center, Durham, NC 27710, USA
5. Department of Pharmacy, Duke University Medical Center, Durham, NC 27710, USA
6. Duke University School of Nursing, Durham, NC 27710, USA; loretta.matters@duke.edu
7. Cecil G. Sheps Center for Health Services Research at University of North Carolina, Chapel Hill, NC 27516, USA; bobkonrad@gmail.com
8. Durham VA Geriatric Research, Education and Clinical Center, Durham, NC 27705, USA
* Correspondence: gwendolen.buhr@duke.edu

Received: 9 August 2019; Accepted: 16 October 2019; Published: 21 October 2019

Abstract: Primary care practices lack the time, expertise, and resources to perform traditional comprehensive geriatric assessment. In particular, they need methods to improve their capacity to identify and care for older adults with complex care needs, such as cognitive impairment. As the US population ages, discovering strategies to address these complex care needs within primary care are urgently needed. This article describes the development of an innovative, team-based model to improve the diagnosis and care of older adults with cognitive impairment in primary care practices. This model was developed through a mentoring process from a team with expertise in geriatrics and quality improvement. Refinement of the existing assessment process performed during routine care allowed patients with cognitive impairment to be identified. The practice team then used a collaborative workflow to connect patients with appropriate community resources. Utilization of these processes led to reduced referrals to the geriatrics specialty clinic, fewer patients presenting in a crisis to the social worker, and greater collaboration and self-efficacy for care of those with cognitive impairment within the practice. Although the model was initially developed to address cognitive impairment, the impact has been applied more broadly to improve the care of older adults with multimorbidity.

Keywords: geriatrics; collaborative practice; geriatric workforce enhancement program; primary care

1. Introduction

The limitations of primary care practices' capacity to care for older adults have been underscored by the Institute of Medicine, which recommended a workforce with enhanced geriatric competence and reimbursement policies that would reward effective models of care for older adults [1]. Further, the World Health Organization has advocated for the development of age friendly primary health centers accessible to older adults, employing healthcare workers well versed in geriatric syndromes and knowledgeable about community resources [2]. More recently, the Institute for Healthcare Improvement (IHI) proposed that all care for older adults be age-friendly, which they have defined as utilizing the 4Ms—What Matters, Medication, Mentation, and Mobility—to make the complex care of older adults more manageable [3].

Diagnosing dementia presents challenges for primary care practices who lack the expertise, time, and resources to perform traditional comprehensive geriatric assessment. Yet, primary care practices are caring for an increasingly older and more complex older adult patient population. In particular, 20% of those older than 65 years have mild cognitive impairment and 14% over 70 years have dementia, yet cognitive impairment is markedly underdiagnosed in primary care [4]. In its traditional form, comprehensive geriatric assessment is an interprofessional and multidimensional process that utilizes the expertise of nurses, physicians, social workers, and other health professionals to evaluate not only physical illness, but also functional status and environmental and social issues, so as to create a plan to optimize wellbeing [5]. Comprehensive geriatric assessment is the ideal process for the diagnosis and care of patients with cognitive impairment. However, it is challenging for most busy primary care practices that care for older people with multimorbidity to employ such a model.

A systematic review of the barriers primary care practices face when diagnosing and managing patients with dementia found that the barriers could be grouped into patient factors, provider factors, and system factors [6]. In particular, the studies found that primary care practices lacked essential support services, including limited access to and knowledge of community resources, lack of access to an interprofessional team to enhance management, and lack of caregiver education and support. In addition, the research found that primary care practices lacked time and sufficient reimbursement to adequately diagnose and manage patients with dementia, as well as a lack of training undermined providers' confidence in making the diagnosis and managing subsequent care. The patient factors included stigma attached to receiving a diagnosis of dementia and delayed presentation of the patient to primary care for memory complaints. This article will describe a process by which an exemplary primary care practice developed an interprofessional and multidimensional process for the care of the older adults with mentoring from a team of geriatric experts. In particular, the practice focused on developing a method to more effectively identify and care for older adults with cognitive impairment.

2. Materials and Methods

The Duke Geriatric Workforce Enhancement Program (Duke-GWEP) was established to develop a healthcare workforce that maximizes patient and family engagement and improves health outcomes for older adults by integrating geriatrics with primary care [7]. To achieve this goal, we recruited primary care practices, and worked with them to create interprofessional geriatric resource teams (GRT) that could serve as a source of expertise in geriatrics and quality improvement (QI) within the practice. Each GRT was unique to the practice, but contained diverse professionals working within the practice—i.e., physicians, nurses, social worker, physician assistants, nurse practitioner, pharmacist, etc. We provided the GRTs a curriculum focused on team building, geriatric knowledge and skills, QI methods, and access to expert consultation and community resources using a hybrid learning model (Figure 1).

Previously, we found that before expecting teams to carry out QI projects, they need to establish a foundation of interprofessional collaborative practice. Therefore, GRT training began with a workshop on interprofessional collaborative practice, based on the Interprofessional Education Collaborative four core competency domains of values and ethics, roles and responsibilities, communication, and teamwork [8]. We emphasized the importance of engaging all team members in shared vision and problem solving using flexible role definitions and encouraging all team members to work at the top of their scope of practice.

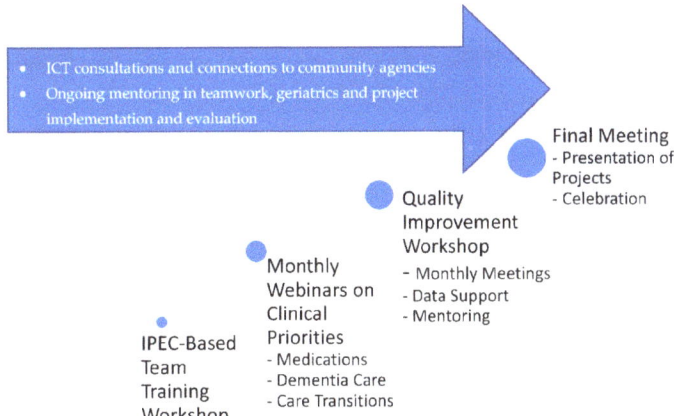

Figure 1. Geriatric Workforce Enhancement Program Primary Care Geriatric Resource Team Training: a year-long commitment to educational programs and process improvement activities. Abbreviations: ICT: Interagency Care Team; IPEC: Interprofessional Education Collaborative.

Throughout the academic year, we held monthly webinars that focused on three clinical priorities specified by the GWEP funding—dementia, medication management, and care transitions—and highlighted local community resources and agencies to help address these issues (Table 1). The webinars were recorded and provided continuing education credit. The GRTs were assigned mentors from the Duke-GWEP team who guided them in choosing QI topics prior to a QI workshop that was held midway through the academic year. We encouraged practices to implement a practice improvement project focused on one of the three priority topics. The QI workshop is based on the IHI model for improvement [9]. We also provided data support and mentoring. We encouraged practices to hold monthly GRT meetings with the GRT members, the Duke-GWEP mentors, and a data support specialist. The data support specialist had expertise in public health research, health communication, project management, IT/data management, and community engagement. At the end of the year all of the GRTs gathered together to present their QI projects.

Table 1. Geriatric resource teams (GRT) webinar topics.

Title	Objectives
Deprescribing	• Explain the process of deprescribing • Assess a patient's need for deprescribing • List at least two services provided by Senior PharmAssist, a community resource that provides financial assistance, medication management, community referrals, and Medicare insurance counseling
Improving Care Transitions	• Define the core principles of high-quality transitions of care • Describe a model for improving transitions in primary care practice • Identify community resources to improve transitions of care
Improving Skilled Nursing Facility (SNF) to Home Care Transitions	• Define the core principles of high-quality transitions of care from SNF to home • Describe a process and model for improving SNF to home transitions that engages teams from facility, health system, community, and primary care practices • Identify a role for options counselors in aiding the transitions process

Table 1. *Cont.*

Title	Objectives
Dementia: Recognition and Initial Assessment	• Describe the scope and impact of dementia • Develop a strategy for improving case recognition of cognitive impairment using questionnaires, structured assessments and specialty referrals • Communicate effectively with older adults and families with suspected cognitive disorders • Identify resources to help seniors and families cope with cognitive problems
Living with Dementia: Safety, Security, and Staying at Home	• Describe the balance between autonomy and safety in caring for people with dementia • List methods for improving safe management of finances and medications • Develop a plan for maintaining home safety • Implement measures to reduce falls among people with dementia
Medication Safety: Preventing Adverse Drug Events and Improving Transition of Care	• Define and classify medication errors and preventable medication related harms • Identify medication related quality measures for various care providers and settings • Identify opportunities to engage community pharmacists in healthcare improvement • Explain the difference between medication therapy management and medication management • List at least 3 community resources for medication management
Accounting for Health Literacy in Primary Care of Older Adults	• Acknowledge that healthcare is complex and problems with understanding and adherence are universal • Describe the association of low health literacy with poor health outcomes • Identify strategies for enhancing communication in practice to optimize a personal experience and outcomes

The Duke-GWEP also offered GRTs access to an Interagency Care Team (ICT): a team of geriatricians, nurse practitioners, and community partners, including clinical pharmacists and social workers who provided virtual consultations via the Electronic Health Record (EHR) for older adults with complex care needs residing in the community. This Duke-GWEP-ICT contacted the patient and family member, did a chart review, and met together to discuss the case and identify resources to help the patient remain at home. A recommendation was subsequently made to the patient and family member and to the providers at the practice.

3. Results

The Duke-GWEP recruited 13 practices in total over the three years, four in year 1, three in year 2, and six in year 3. To illustrate how comprehensive geriatric assessment principles are implemented in primary care, we present as a case one of the primary care practices from the first of three GRT cohorts.

Example GRT at the Duke Outpatient Clinic (DOC)

The DOC is the major internal medicine resident teaching clinic for Duke University Medical Center, where the physician faculty and interprofessional staff recognized the challenge of caring for older adults. The clinic serves a medically and socially complex group of 4500 patients, with an average age of 62 years, many of whom are under- or uninsured. The clinic employs an interprofessional team including a licensed clinical social worker who also functions as a behavioral health specialist, a Clinical Pharmacist Practitioner, registered nurses, certified medical assistants (CMA), attending physicians, and more than 70 internal medicine residents. The DOC GRT members included the licensed clinical social worker, behavioral health specialist, Clinical Pharmacist Practitioner, attending physician and clinic medical director, and a registered nurse.

Prior to forming the GRT, there was neither a systematic approach to identify patients with cognitive impairment nor a routine process to connect patients with dementia and their caregivers to needed community resources. Barriers identified by clinic staff included a lack of expertise in the diagnosis and management of patients with cognitive impairment and a lack of time. Consequently, the evaluation of cognitive impairment often did not happen until a crisis occurred, and the default response was to refer to the geriatric specialty clinic for comprehensive geriatric assessment. Timely access to this resource was hampered by a wait time of several months to obtain an appointment, and the need to visit the large medical center across town, which resulted in missed appointments. Because many patient and family crises involved an immediate need for placement, this sometimes resulted in a hospital admission for the patient.

During the workshops, the DOC team developed both a formal vision statement and QI aim. Vision statement: "Partner with the Duke-GWEP to foster educational initiatives, interdisciplinary care teams, and collaboration with community resources to improve the care of older adult patients and their loved ones-with a specific focus on cognitive impairment." QI project aim: "Develop and implement an interdisciplinary approach to improve care of patients and families affected by cognitive impairment."

After developing the vision and aim statements, the clinic's first step was workflow development, so as to screen for and diagnose cognitive impairment and clarify a process for caring for the patient once cognitive impairment was recognized. The GRT met monthly with their interprofessional team and Duke-GWEP mentors to systematically work through developing care processes to support the workflow, identify gaps, and provide additional training. The initial screening was incorporated into an ongoing project to screen for problems of social determinants of health. The team added a question to the existing screening form—"In the last two months, have you or your family had concerns about your memory or thinking?" In response to a positive answer, cognitive evaluation was then initiated using the Mini-Cog [10] performed by the CMA or the Montreal Cognitive Assessment tool (MoCA) [11] performed by the social worker, as well as for patients with concerns identified by the medical team. As the project continued, requests for cognitive evaluation began to increase from once every few months to a few times a week as providers became more aware of the clinical indicators of cognitive impairment.

The GRT developed a second workflow to guide the next steps after cognitive impairment was identified. The team obtained collateral history, performed further medical work up and treatment, documented cognitive impairment on the problem list within the EHR, and then counselled the patient and family on the diagnosis and treatment plan. An important aspect of the treatment plan was linking the patient and their caregivers to the appropriate community resources such as caregiver support programs. As cognitive impairment is now being identified earlier in the trajectory of illness, and not necessarily in conjunction with a crisis, there has been a resultant dramatic decrease in both requests for emergency placement for patients and referrals to the geriatric specialty clinic (Figure 2). The clinic is now only referring their most complex patients who can be seen more promptly since the less complex patients are managed within the primary care practice.

As part of their new process for screening, assessing, and providing care for patients with cognitive impairment, the clinic created a patient list of those with identified cognitive impairment to ensure that some of the most vulnerable patients received the services they needed. For example, they used that list to take a more proactive role in reviewing the advance care planning (ACP) needs and prioritizing these patients for ACP visits [12].

Although the model was developed to address cognitive impairment, the impact has been greater, expanding to focus on older adults with multimorbidity. The model continues to evolve and grow as other needs are uncovered. Beginning in quarter 3 of 2018, the team implemented an internal process for interdisciplinary review of complex patients, using a population health approach in which patients were identified for review by the clinical social workers based on presence of dementia and multimorbidity. The GRT modeled their processes after the Duke-GWEP's ICT and received consultation from the Duke-GWEP nurse practitioner who developed the ICT systems. Specifically, the clinical social worker and clinical pharmacist practitioner completed a thorough review of issues regarding cognition, medication access, medication management, disease management, advance care planning, social determinants of health, labs, behavioral health/social isolation, personal/home safety, insurance/access to care, and transitions of care. The review was documented in the EHR and reviewed with the entire team including physicians and geriatrics consultants at monthly meetings.

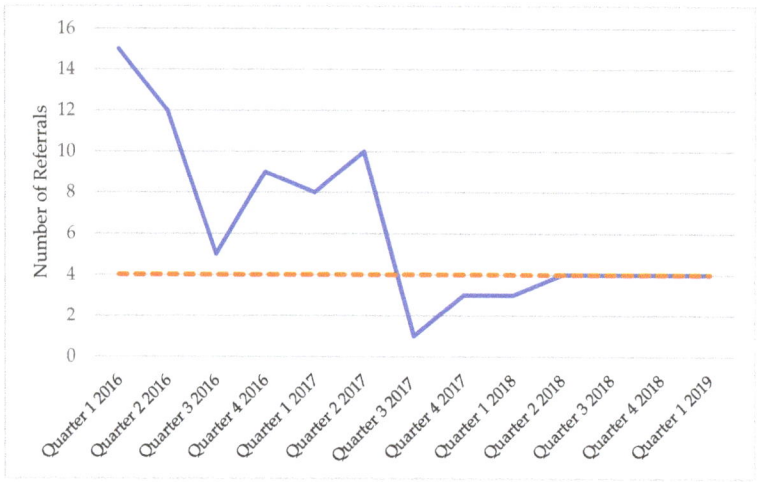

Figure 2. Number of referrals to the geriatric specialty clinic from the beginning of the project. The orange dotted line indicates the median.

Case Studies

The following case studies serve to illustrate how developing a GRT in a primary care practice enhances the capacity for conducting comprehensive geriatric assessment within primary care.

Case 1: An 88-year-old female with multiple medical problems, including recurrent GI bleeding, COPD, glaucoma, cachexia, and osteoarthritis, was abruptly left without a caregiver when her son unexpectedly died. She experienced worsening mental status and mood in the last year of her life, including an episode of delirium. Prior to establishing the GRT, this type of patient would have received a referral to the geriatrics clinic for comprehensive geriatric assessment. Instead, the primary care practice was able to manage the patient's complex needs without a geriatrics referral. The GRT's enhanced expertise in evaluation of her cognitive disturbance, enhanced teamwork processes, and awareness of community resources led to a timely referral to adult protective services and establishment of a new healthcare power of attorney (HCPOA) to replace her son who had recently died. Soon after, the patient experienced a serious health crisis. Her HCPOA was able to advocate effectively due to the work that had been done, and the patient was transferred to an inpatient hospice, where she died while receiving comfort care, in accordance with her wishes.

Case 2: At an acute care visit, a 63-year-old patient complained of word-finding and trouble remembering her medications. Prior to forming a GRT, the provider would have noted the concerns and advised that the patient follow-up with her primary care provider (PCP), and if the complaint persisted, a referral to the geriatrics specialty clinic would have occurred. Instead, the provider referred the patient to the GRT social worker, who was already embedded in the clinic, and able to administer the MoCA. The patient's score was 22 out of 30; however, most of the points missed were in executive function, not memory or attention. So, the social worker, recognizing that depression can present atypically in older adults, administered a depression screen. The patient tearfully reported that her mother had died 3 years ago last week, and admitted that she has not slept well since her mother passed away, getting on average about 3 h of sleep a night. The PHQ-9 results were 19 out of 26, and after declining counseling, the patient accepted pharmacotherapy for her depression. Even though the primary diagnosis was depression, not dementia, the presence of the GRT and related protocols for cognitive impairment improved teamwork and access to staff with geriatrics expertise that, in turn, supported the diagnosis and treatment of depression which had previously been undetected.

4. Discussion

The barriers to the diagnosis of dementia in primary care are myriad and include provider factors, patient factors, and system factors. The GRT effectively addressed most of these barriers. Specifically, the practice was provided with training and mentorship to increase the knowledge of the providers in the identification, evaluation and management of cognitive impairment. In addition, much attention was given to linking patients and their families to community resources to support them in their homes. Further, patients were universally screened for memory concerns, addressing the barrier of delayed presentation. The time constraints and reimbursement issues remain challenging [13], but the team is better positioned to utilize all members of the interprofessional team to address some of these barriers. The GRT example and case studies illustrate effective collaborative care for patients with complex care needs, including dementia, in primary care. The members of the GRT engaged in shared problem solving; rather than a workflow that relied on one profession to identify and care for the older adult, flexible role definitions were developed that allow each profession to work at the top of their scope of practice (Figure 3).

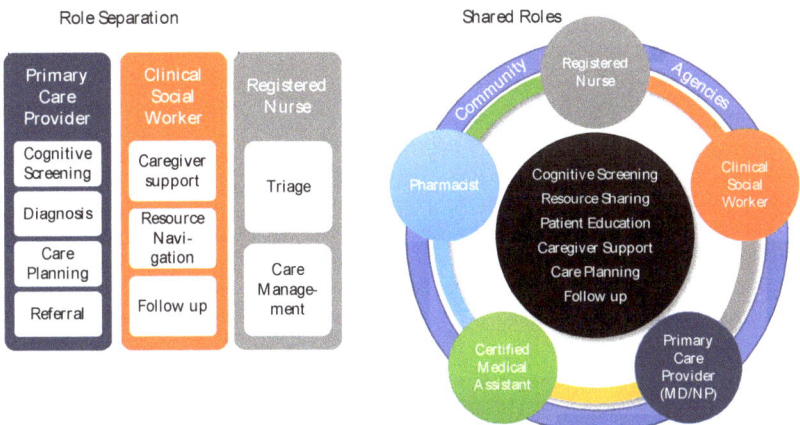

Figure 3. Redefining Roles and Workflow in Geriatric Primary Care before and after the establishment of a GRT.

Although not all of the team members received GRT training, the effects spread to all team members. As a result of the Duke-GWEP, the CMAs received additional geriatric training from the Duke Nurses Improving Care for Healthsystem Elders (Duke-NICHE) program [14], and for subsequent GRTs similar training was offered upfront. The Duke-GWEP training resulted in enhanced trust and confidence especially between the physicians and non-physician team members to identify and address geriatric issues. The social worker previously was brought in only during a crisis and the pharmacist was not involved. Now the pharmacist is involved in deprescribing and the social worker helps when mild cognitive impairment is identified, and an EHR-based patient list for all patients in the practice with cognitive impairment has been established so that their care needs can be anticipated and managed proactively. The CMAs are now more often included in the team discussions regarding patients and are viewed by the providers as key members of the team, resulting in empowerment and a greater sense of purpose or meaning. The practice learned from the Duke-GWEP virtual consultations performed by the ICT and was able to adopt these strategies for resource referrals to help other patients with similar problems—fall prevention, medication recommendations, and community resources.

Many programs strive to improve the care of older adults in primary care with system changes or processes with variable degrees of success [15,16]. The GRT program was unique in that there was an emphasis on team formation and webinars on geriatric principles and community resources coupled with mentoring by geriatric experts.

This example GRT from the DOC has applicability to teaching clinics in other academic health centers. As trainees rotate through these clinics that model interprofessional collaborative practice and team-based care, we expect to see improved uptake of processes that expand capacity through more effective teamwork. Team-based care that includes a variety of disciplines working to the top of their scope of practice and with expanded geriatric competency can achieve improved care of older adults without higher costs [17]. Furthermore, we believe that with the current structure of Medicare reimbursement, mentored comprehensive geriatric assessment is possible within primary care practices. Recognizing changes in cognition is a required part of the Medicare Annual Wellness Visit (G0438, G0439). As of January of 2018, Medicare provides reimbursement to providers for a comprehensive clinical visit for patients with dementia, resulting in a written care plan (CPT code 99483). This code requires an independent historian; a multidimensional assessment that includes cognition, function, and safety; evaluation of neuropsychiatric and behavioral symptoms; review and reconciliation of medications; and assessment of the needs of the patient's caregiver. These additional billing codes provide reimbursement for practitioners for the additional time that is required in the care of these patients.

The model of shared roles allows for flexibility in the role definitions. The key is to engage all team members in shared problem solving and to make sure all of the team members are working at the top of their scope of practice. In addition, linkages with community resources are critical, as well as enhanced training in geriatrics. This example GRT illustrates sustainability since the initial training occurred over three years ago, and the practice has developed systems to sustain the program despite only one year of intensive support from the Duke-GWEP. By focusing on team formation and interprofessional collaborative practice, the teams were equipped to continue their work. We are investigating models to continue to support primary care practices in their care of older adults. This can occur through the accountable care organization or through various e-consult or telehealth programs. Without GWEP funding, teams can obtain training on geriatric care principles, QI, and interprofessional collaborative practice through a variety of professional development opportunities and organizations, such as IPEC, American Geriatric Society, and the IHI age-friendly health systems resources.

Author Contributions: Conceptualization, E.M., J.D., H.C., L.B., and C.D.; methodology, T.K., G.B., E.M., and M.H.; formal analysis, C.D. and G.B.; investigation, J.D., H.C., E.N., L.B., E.M., and C.D.; data curation, C.D.; writing—original draft preparation, G.B.; writing—review and editing, L.B., J.D., G.B., C.D., E.N., H.C., and T.K., L.P., E.M., M.H.; visualization, L.P., G.B., C.D., M.H., and E.M.; supervision, M.H., G.B.; funding acquisition, E.M., M.H., and L.M.

Funding: This research was funded by a U.S. Bureau of Health Professions Health Resources and Services Administration (HRSA) Geriatric Workforce Enhancement Program (GWEP) grant (U1QHP28708).

Conflicts of Interest: The authors declare no conflicts of interest.

References

1. Institute of Medicine (IOM). *Retooling for an Aging America: Building the Health Care Workforce*; The National Academies Press: Washington, DC, USA, 2008.
2. World Health Organization. Age-friendly Primary Health Care Centres Toolkit. 2008. Available online: https://www.who.int/ageing/publications/AF_PHC_Centretoolkit.pdf (accessed on 12 July 2019).

3. Age-Friendly Health Systems: Guide to Using the 4Ms in the Care of Older Adults. April 2019. Available online: http://www.ihi.org/Engage/Initiatives/Age-Friendly-Health-Systems/Documents/IHIAgeFriendlyHealthSystems_GuidetoUsing4MsCare.pdf (accessed on 12 July 2019).
4. Alzheimer's Association. 2019 Alzheimer's Disease Facts and Figures. *Alzheimers Dement.* **2019**, *15*, 321–387. [CrossRef]
5. Rubenstein, L.Z.; Stuck, A.E.; Siu, A.L.; Wieland, D. Impacts of Geriatric Evaluation and Management Programs on defined Outcomes: Overview of the Evidence. *J. Am. Geriat. Soc.* **1991**, *39*, 8S–16S. [CrossRef] [PubMed]
6. Koch, T.; Iliffe, S.; EVIDEM-ED Project. Rapid appraisal of barriers to the diagnosis and management of patients with dementia in primary care: A systematic review. *BMC Fam. Pract.* **2010**, *11*, 52. [CrossRef] [PubMed]
7. Health Resources and Services Administration. Geriatric Workforce Enhancement Program. 8 November 2018. Available online: https://bhw.hrsa.gov/fundingopportunities/default.aspx?id=4c8ee9ff-617a-495e-ae78-917847db86a9 (accessed on 21 September 2019).
8. Interprofessional Education Collaborative Expert Panel. *Core Competencies for Interprofessional Collaborative Practice: Report of an Expert Panel*; Interprofessional Education Collaborative: Washington, DC, USA, 2011.
9. Ogrinc, G.S.; Headrick, L.A.; Moore, S.M.; Barton, A.J.; Dolansky, M.A.; Madigosky, W.S. *Fundamentals of Health Care Improvement: A Guide to Improving Your Patients' Care*, 2nd ed.; The Joint Commission and the Institute for Healthcare Improvement: Oakbrook Terrace, IL, USA, 2012.
10. Borson, S.; Scanlan, J.; Brush, M.; Vitaliano, P.; Dokmak, A. The Mini-Cog: A cognitive 'vital signs' measure for dementia screening in multi-lingual elderly. *Int. J. Geriatr. Psychiatry* **2000**, *15*, 1021–1027. [CrossRef]
11. Razak, M.A.; Ahmad, N.A.; Chan, Y.Y.; Kasim, N.M.; Yusof, M.; Ghani, M.A.; Omar, M.; Abd Aziz, F.A.; Jamaluddin, R. Validity of screening tools for dementia and mild cognitive impairment among the elderly in primary health care: A systematic review. *Public Health* **2019**, *169*, 84–92. [CrossRef] [PubMed]
12. Frequently Asked Questions about Billing the Physician Fee Schedule for Advance Care Planning Services. July 2016. Available online: https://www.cms.gov/Medicare/Medicare-Fee-for-Service-Payment/PhysicianFeeSched/Downloads/FAQ-Advance-Care-Planning.pdf (accessed on 3 August 2019).
13. Boustani, M.; Alder, C.A.; Solid, C.A.; Reuben, D. An Alternative Payment Model to Support Widespread Use of Collaborative Dementia Care Models. *Health Aff.* **2019**, *38*, 54–59. [CrossRef] [PubMed]
14. Hendrix, C.C.; Matters, L.; West, Y.; Stewart, B.; McConnell, E.S. The Duke-NICHE program: An academic-practice collaboration to enhance geriatric nursing care. *Nurs. Outlook* **2011**, *59*, 149–157. [CrossRef] [PubMed]
15. Giuliante, M.M.; Greenberg, S.A.; McDonald, M.V.; Squires, A.; Moore, R.; Cortes, T.A. Geriatric Interdisciplinary Team Training 2.0: A collaborative team-based approach to delivering care. *J. Interprof. Care* **2018**, *32*, 629–633. [CrossRef] [PubMed]
16. Elliott, J.; Stolee, P.; Boscart, V.; Giangregorio, L.; Heckman, G. Coordinating care for older adults in primary care settings: Understanding the current context. *BMC Fam. Pract.* **2018**, *19*, 137. [CrossRef] [PubMed]
17. Kunik, M.E.; Mills, W.L.; Amspoker, A.B.; Cully, J.A.; Kraus-Schuman, C.; Stanley, M.; Wilson, N.L. Expanding the geriatric mental health workforce through utilization of non-licensed providers. *Aging Ment. Health* **2017**, *21*, 954–960. [CrossRef] [PubMed]

© 2019 by the authors. Licensee MDPI, Basel, Switzerland. This article is an open access article distributed under the terms and conditions of the Creative Commons Attribution (CC BY) license (http://creativecommons.org/licenses/by/4.0/).

MDPI
St. Alban-Anlage 66
4052 Basel
Switzerland
Tel. +41 61 683 77 34
Fax +41 61 302 89 18
www.mdpi.com

Geriatrics Editorial Office
E-mail: geriatrics@mdpi.com
www.mdpi.com/journal/geriatrics

www.ingramcontent.com/pod-product-compliance
Lightning Source LLC
LaVergne TN
LVHW070606100526
838202LV00012B/581